PUT THAT FRIED CHICKEN DOWN

FIVE SIMPLE STEPS FOR SOUTHERNERS TO JUMPSTART THEIR HEALTH JOURNEY

DR. JENNIFER WHITMON

Paperback: 978-1-64746-336-6
Hardback: 978-1-64746-337-3
Ebook: 978-1-64746-338-0

Library of Congress Control Number: 2020911276

Scripture quotations are taken from the King James Version of the Holy Bible. The author italicized all Bible verses as a personal choice.

This book contains the opinions and ideas of its author. They are solely for informational and educational purposes and should not be regarded as a substitute for professional medical treatment. The nature of your body's health condition is complex and unique to you. Therefore, you should consult a health professional before you begin any new exercise, nutrition, or supplementation program or if you have questions about your health. Neither the author nor the publisher shall be liable or responsible for any medical outcomes that may occur arising from any information or suggestions in this book.

The statements in this book about consumable products or food have not been evaluated by the Food and Drug Administration. The publisher is not responsible for your specific health or allergy needs that may require medical supervision. The publisher and author are not responsible for any adverse reactions to the consumption of food or products that have been suggested in this book.

Dedication

In memory of my parents, Antoinette and Junior, who
always supported and guided me to excel in my endeavors.
And in honor of my cousin and family mentor, Charles, who
offered me encouragement and support in my educational
and business pursuits. And to my readers, I hope you find
this book to be good for your body and soul.

Contents

Part 2 If the Creek Don't Rise: Making Better Choices

Part 3 Who Are Your People? Accountability Is the Key to Success

Appendices

Acknowledgments

I would like to thank my patient and loving husband, John, who was my first client and stimulus for the development of the five steps in this book. Thank you for your love and support throughout the writing process.

To my precious daughter, Joie, who implemented the five steps in the book and understands the importance of maintaining good health through diet and exercise. I am proud of you.

I extend special thanks to my cousin, Carrie who listened to me talk about the book from its inception and helped me to refine the five steps in the book and pushed me to finish.

To my sisters, Karen and Adrianne, thank you both for moving back to the South and continually helping me to stay motivated to complete this book.

To my mother-in law, Yvonne, for always encouraging me and keeping me focused.

To my friends, Bishop Lewis, Clarietha, and Betty, thank you for your prayers and support for the success of the book.

Special thanks to my beta readers, my friend, Saundra who gave me innovative business strategies after the review of the book, and my cousin, Shelia who graciously read the book and gave me practical suggestions for making the book better, and my longtime friend, Lydia, who took the time to provide a thorough scientific and health information review of the book.

Introduction

Whether therefore ye eat, or drink, or whatsoever ye do,
do all to the glory of God.

—1 Corinthians 10:31

Yes, you read the title correctly. *Put That Fried Chicken Down: Five Simple Steps for Southerners to Jumpstart Their Health Journey.* This book is not a condemnation of fried chicken or Southerners. It is about my experiences growing up in the wonderful South eating fried chicken, and it is about my health journey and the five simple steps that will inspire you to jumpstart *your* health journey.

Churches and Fried Chicken.

I was raised in a small town in Alabama in the Bible Belt, the region in the South where church attendance is historically higher. In this region, there are hundreds of churches, including multiple churches in single neighborhoods. I went to church most Sundays and was familiar with Southern church culture. My town was full of Southern hospitality with a strong community and churches. Southern hospitality meant everyone was welcomed at all events. If no one knew you, they might have asked, "Are you from around here?" Ultimately, they treated you like family. A strong community meant people knew each other and were willing to help neighbors as well as strangers. I remember church and community events held at our small Baptist church like anniversaries and events like weddings, funerals, and graduation dinners. At every event, the Pastor and *fried chicken* were present. Not only did the pastor lead worship service on Sundays, which required long hours of preparation during the week, but he prayed for parishioners and guests during those worship services and gave words of encouragement. He also greeted everyone in the building. Unfortunately, pastors and other men and women of the clergy tend to take care of others and not take care of themselves, physically, emotionally or mentally.[1] The information presented in this book is applicable to pastors, clergy, lay leaders, or anyone who serves others while neglecting their needs in the process.

At church events, the most popular food item was fried chicken. The standard fried chicken meal included macaroni and cheese, collard greens or other green vegetables seasoned with fatty meat, cornbread, sweet tea, and pound cake. Please don't get me wrong—I loved these foods as much as the next person, but we ate these foods during special occasions, and special occasions were in abundance. In the South, one of the most important aspects of a gathering was the food.

When I moved to another Southern state as a young adult, I realized that Southerners stick to the traditions they love like college football and tailgating, pickup trucks, and backyard parties. And when it came to food, Southerners held on even stronger to traditions by eating foods such as buttermilk biscuits and sausage gravy, peach cobbler, fatback, hogshead cheese, and grilled meat with BBQ sauce. When I attended another Southern church, I had the same types of meals at that church and for special dinners with friends and other social occasions. Over the years, I noticed my weight, blood pressure, and clothing size all increased. I learned first-hand what I put on my plate was directly linked to the status of my health.

Southerners usually stick to one eating pattern—fried and fatty foods, food with added fats, eggs, sugary drinks, and processed meats such as bacon, ham, and organ meats. One study found that people who eat this traditional Southern eating pattern had an increased risk of developing coronary heart disease, which increases the risk for heart attack or stroke. People who ate the Southern eating pattern foods were also more likely to have diabetes and hypertension.[2] When we frequently eat processed foods and foods full of bad fats and sugars, we are setting ourselves up for poor health.

Not only is the South referred to as the Bible Belt, but over the last ten years, it has been deemed the Obesity Belt[3], and the Diabetes Belt[4] because of unusually high incidences of obesity, diabetes, and other forms of cardiovascular disease. It includes Southern states like Alabama, Georgia, Kentucky, Louisiana, Mississippi, North Carolina, South Carolina, and Tennessee. Chronic diseases are linked to dietary patterns and other factors not as easy to change such as poverty, race, and access to healthcare. The reason I began this book was to bring awareness to the health conditions associated with the Southern eating pattern.

If I don't follow the Southern eating pattern, then what do I eat?

The second reason I wrote the book was to simplify information about foods and healthy eating to empower you to make better choices. Research studies about food are contradictory, which makes it difficult to understand how to change your diet. On any given year, a study shows up about an unhealthy food group, but within the next few years, another study disproves what the previous study concluded. Information overload causes a panic, and you ask health-related questions. For example, I met a Southern friend for lunch who I had not seen in years. At lunch, we began to discuss my health coaching practice and healthy food choices. She mentioned she did not know how to eat healthy, and she was consumed with changing food information. She began to ask a plethora of questions such as "Can I eat a banana? If so, what time of the day? Do I eat the egg yolk or the egg white? What are good carbs? And what are bad carbs?" After our lunch, I sent her a one-page newsletter with healthy food choices and practical tips. The next week I did the same. After writing the one-page newsletter for the third week, I realized I could write a book using this knowledge. I knew many people from the South did not know the basics of eating healthy, so overwhelm and confusion sets in with all the health and nutrition information they see and read.

Advertisers spend an exuberant amount of money to get you to go out and buy what you see in the media. There is no exception in the food industry. The Southern eating pattern and ultraprocessed fast food is a recipe for a health crisis. When you select food with excess sugar, sodium, and fat, your taste buds and brains are overstimulated, which causes healthy whole foods to taste bland. A solution to this is to retrain your taste buds. It is wise to read nutrition facts labels and the ingredient lists of your foods because it gives you the power to decide what and how much goes in your body and to make informed choices.

Food is culture and tradition for Southerners. Most of your eating patterns began in childhood. Therefore, you must examine your eating patterns and what you learned about your food choices. If your food choices and eating patterns are risk factors for chronic disease and some diseases are a matter of life and death, you might have to relearn what and how to eat.

The third reason I wrote the book is to remind you that we must be accountable to each other. I will use my education and experience as a certified health coach and *Southerner* to show it is not only possible to easily eat healthier, but it does not have to be confusing. As the old saying goes, "If we know better, we do better." It is time to put your faith into action as it relates to diet, which affects our health. God wants you to have a life of abundance spiritually, emotionally, financially, and physically. You cannot always change your circumstances, but you can change your behavior. Eating patterns are behavioral choices.

You are beginning the first phase of the process—awareness of the problems. The information in this book has five simple steps that are easy to understand and implement. You owe it to yourself to live your best life, which means you look good, feel better, and have increased energy.

PART 1

I Was Born at Night but Not Last Night!

Awareness

1

Bless Your Heart

Health Problems Associated with the Southern Diet

What? know ye not that your body is the temple of the Holy Ghost which is in you, which ye have of God and ye are not your own. For we are bought with a price: therefore, glorify God in your body, and in your spirit, which are God's.

—1 Corinthians 6:19-20

My family's medical history is no different than other families from the South. Family members suffer from obesity and have died of heart disease, stroke, and cancer. My father developed type 2 diabetes in his sixties. He was not overweight when he was diagnosed but had complications which led to amputation of two toes. We think my father had symptoms of diabetes long before he was diagnosed. My father did not die of diabetes or its complications, but he died from lung cancer associated with smoking.

Unfortunately, he smoked for many years and grew up in an era when smoking was the norm, but the long-term health effects were unknown, ignored, or not acknowledged. My mother was also diagnosed with diabetes in her sixties. She controlled her condition with medication, but she died at the age of sixty-seven, two years after diagnosis and complications of multiple myeloma. At the time, it was a rare form of cancer. Both of my parents passed at the age of sixty-seven, two years apart. My daughter was an infant when my father passed and was two years old when my mother passed. For a while, I feared I might die from some disease at the age of sixty-seven, but after praying about that fear, God reminded me fear does not come from Him. 2 Timothy 1:7 states, *"For God hath not given us the spirit of fear; but of power, and of love, and of a sound mind."* He quickly reminded me that my paternal great grandmother lived to be 102 years old.

In church, you learned your bodies are medical miracles. The systems of your body work together perfectly. God encourages you to care for your bodies as it is described in 1 Corinthians 6:19. *"What? know ye not that your body is the temple of the Holy Ghost, which is in you, which ye have of God, and ye are not your own?"* Eating healthier is one of the physical counterparts to maintaining your temples in service to the Lord, and this helps you bring His kingdom to earth. For example, we hear a lot about detoxing programs. God designed your bodies to naturally detox through organs within your bodies. Here are two examples. Your liver is an organ with many roles, and one of these roles is to help detoxify your bodies. The liver acts as a filter to make sure toxins (viruses, bacteria, drugs, harmful chemicals, alcohol) are removed from the blood. Because the liver has many functions, it can regenerate itself if it is not damaged. God knew what He was doing when He so meticulously designed your bodies! The kidneys are also detoxifying organs. Two roles the kidneys play are to regulate fluid and electrolytes (calcium, sodium, potassium) balances in the body and filter the blood. It is possible to badly damage the kidneys with years of toxin overloads such as medications or alcohol. Over time, poor diets or other factors may cause your organs to work harder, which results in disease. God created your bodies to fight off diseases with organs that can help to detoxify your bodies. The liver and kidneys are two examples of these types of organs, but there may be an interruption to natural defenses when chronic diseases occur. In this chapter, we will discuss common chronic diseases that may be delayed, prevented, or managed through diet and lifestyle changes.

Chronic diseases are health conditions that last more than one year and require treatment or monitoring. Six out of ten Americans suffer from one chronic disease and four out of ten suffer from two or more chronic diseases.[1] Studies show that more than half of older adults have three or more chronic diseases occurring at the same time.[2] More than 66% of deaths are caused by chronic diseases, heart disease, cancer, stroke, chronic pulmonary disease, and diabetes. Chronic diseases are responsible for seven out of ten deaths in the U.S. killing more than 1.7 million people each year with more than 75% of the two trillion dollars was spent on chronic diseases in public and private healthcare costs.[3, 4, 5]

As you age, it is important to make good choices regarding your health because your bodies change, and you need to prepare for these changes. One study shows that individuals, specifically African Americans, are living longer but developing chronic diseases at an earlier age.[6] As this number increases, more people will enter the hospital and may suffer with a long-term disability, increasing life's challenges, and perhaps even resulting in death.

Obesity plays a factor in chronic diseases. Some medical experts consider obesity to be a chronic disease, but others do not agree. Even though there are factors associated with obesity—genetics, underlying diseases, and medication—for purposes of this book, we will not define obesity as a chronic disease. Other causes of obesity are physical inactivity, poor diet, and overeating. Obesity refers to your body mass index (BMI). It is a term to describe the amount of fat in the body. A high BMI or obesity increases your risk of health problems. A healthcare professional can help to determine your BMI ranges and whether you are obese or overweight. *Being over-weight* means that you have extra body fat or muscle.

A BMI of 30 or higher means that you are obese.[7]
- If your BMI is 18.5 to <25, it is within the normal range.
- If your BMI is 25.0 to <30, it is within the overweight range.
- If your BMI is 30.0 or higher, it is within the obese range.

Obesity is also further subdivided:
- Class 1: BMI of 30 to <35
- Class 2: BMI of 35 to <40
- Class 3: BMI of 40 or higher. This class is considered extreme of severe types of obesity.

According to a 2016 study, there are over 100 million people (adults and children) in the United States who have obesity or severe obesity[8]. The number of people living with obesity in America is increasing and particularly for individuals living in some southern states.[9] Obesity increases the risk for health problems such as high blood pressure, type 2 diabetes, heart disease, kidney disease, arthritis, sleep apnea, liver disease, gallbladder disease, stroke, and certain types of cancer. Let's further explore three of these chronic diseases: heart disease, hypertension, and diabetes.

Heart Disease

As of 2017, heart disease was the leading cause of death for both men and women in the US [10] particularly in Southern states.[11] Heart disease refers to conditions or irregularities of the heart. Cardiovascular disease refers to not only issues of the heart but also blood vessels and the circulatory system. The most common type of heart disease may lead to a heart attack and is called coronary artery disease. Coronary artery disease means there is a problem with blood flow to the heart. Decreased blood flow to the heart causes a heart attack. There are many cardiovascular diseases including hardened arteries, an enlarged heart, heart failure, heart attack, stroke, aneurysm, peripheral artery disease, and sudden cardiac arrest. Other heart conditions exist and have a range of causes, symptoms, and treatments.

A physician diagnoses heart disease. It depends on your medical or family history and your symptoms. Some procedures may include listening to your heart sounds and heart rate, checking your blood pressure or blood tests (cholesterol), electrocardiograms (ECGs), stress tests, or a variety of X-rays or scans.

Risk factors for the conditions are age, race, sex, high blood pressure, obesity, smoking, high cholesterol, diabetes, and a sedentary lifestyle. Family history is another important risk factor. As you age, it is even more important to try to live a healthy lifestyle because you cannot change some risk factors like age, sex, and race. Some types of heart disease are preventable through diet and lifestyle changes. If diagnosed in time and the illness is not too bad, some types of heart disease are manageable. Prevention of heart disease includes having a healthy cholesterol and blood pressure, quitting smoking, and maintaining a healthy weight by eating healthy and exercising. There are some things that you cannot change such as genetics or race, but you can change your diet and lifestyle.

Hypertension

Hypertension or high blood pressure (HBP) is when the force of blood flowing through your artery walls is consistently too high. Constant high blood pressure can damage your arteries and heart. According to the American Heart Association (AHA), HBP affects one in three Americans, 103 million people in America.[12] According to the AHA, from 2005-2015, the actual number of deaths caused by HBP increased 37.5%.[13]

Blood pressure is a measurement of two numbers. The top number refers to systolic pressure, and the bottom number refers to diastolic blood pressure. Systolic pressure is the force when the heart contracts and pumps blood from the chambers of the heart. Diastolic pressure is pressure in your arteries when your heart rests between beats. If you have HBP, your heart works harder and can be damaged because of the increased pressure in your arteries and blood vessels, which may lead to other conditions. In 2017, the guidelines for HBP were changed by the American College of Cardiology (ACC) and AHA. In the past, high blood pressure was determined to be 140 systolic over 90 diastolic. The new guidelines for high blood pressure are 130/80. These guidelines eliminated the category of prehypertension and increased the number of people diagnosed with high blood pressure. These guidelines also determined that high blood pressure should be treated earlier with lifestyle changes and for some patients with medication.[14,15]

The New Blood Pressure Stages

Blood Pressure Category	Systolic mm Hg (upper #)	Diastolic mm Hg (lower #)
Normal	Less than 120 and	Less than 80
Elevation	120-129 and	Less than 80
High Blood Pressure (Hypertension) Stage 1	130-139 or	80-89
High Blood Pressure (Hypertension) Stage 2	140 or higher or	90 or higher
Hypertensive Crisis (Seek Emergency care)	Higher Than 180 and/or	Higher than 120

Rates of HBP have been prevalent in individuals in the South and especially for African Americans and some reports link HBP to a Southern diet with processed meat, fried foods, organ meats, added fats, high dairy foods, sugar sweetened beverages and breads.[16]

HBP may develop over many years without cause. This is primary hypertension.

Secondary hypertension is due to an underlying health condition. Some conditions lead to secondary hypertension like sleep apnea, kidney, thyroid, and adrenal gland issues.

High blood pressure is called the "silent killer" because it has no obvious warning signs or symptoms to indicate your blood pressure is high or extremely high. Undiagnosed or uncontrolled HBP can lead to many health issues such as heart disease, heart attack, stroke, aneurysms, and kidney failure.

Some risk factors for HBP include age, race, family history, smoking, obesity, being physically inactive, high sodium, low potassium in your diet, other chronic conditions, and stress. Eating a healthy diet, getting regular exercise, maintaining a healthy weight, managing stress, and not smoking are some ways to prevent HBP. If diagnosed with HBP and asked to take HBP medication, please be sure to take medication as prescribed. Uncontrolled HBP may cause damage to the heart and to other organs and even death.

Diabetes

Diabetes is a metabolic disorder in which blood sugar or glucose levels in the body remain high. The body is unable to regulate the amount of glucose (sugar) in the blood. Diabetes can cause serious complications and premature death. There are two types of diabetes, type 1, and type 2.

Type 1 diabetes usually begins in children and young people under the age of thirty. In this type of diabetes, a person cannot make the insulin their body needs. The body's immune system destroys the cells in the pancreas that make insulin. Insulin needs to be injected into the body to maintain sugar levels. Type 1 diabetes is commonly found in children, but some adults are diagnosed with it too.

Type 2 diabetes, also called adult onset diabetes, is the most common type of diabetes. In this form of diabetes, some insulin is still being produced but not enough to properly control blood sugar levels. Going forward, we will focus on type 2 diabetes. According to the CDC, 30.3 million people in the United States have diabetes, which is 1 in 4 Americans. More than seven million are undiagnosed. Eighty-four million adults have pre-diabetes, which is one in two people (every other adult we meet). Adults sixty-five and older make up 23.1 million cases of prediabetes.[17] Pre-diabetes is a condition that could lead to type 2 diabetes within five years.

Pre-diabetic individuals are also at risk for developing heart disease and stroke. In the early 2010s, states in the Southern US were deemed the "Diabetes Belt" because of the high rates of diabetes due to obesity and physical inactivity.[18]

Symptoms of diabetes may develop over time. Unfortunately, some individuals have diabetes and do not know it. Symptoms include:

- Increased thirst
- Frequent urination
- Increased hunger
- Frequent infections
- Fatigue
- Weight loss
- Blurred vision

When blood glucose levels are repeatedly high, serious damage can occur in many organs/areas of your body. Complications from diabetes may include heart disease, stroke, end-stage kidney disease, blindness, amputations, and neuropathy.

There is a strong correlation between diabetes and heart disease. Individuals with diabetes are at high risk for heart disease. High blood sugar levels for long periods of time lead to damaged nerves and blood vessels, which may lead to heart disease and stroke. Type 2 diabetes accelerates and intensifies hardening of the arteries because high blood sugar levels cause additional damage to arterial walls and make the blood thick and sticky. This further impairs circulation and places an extra burden on the heart. The direct relationship between heart disease and diabetes is serious and should not be taken lightly. If one has additional risk factors such as obesity, smoking, and high blood pressure, then the chances for heart disease increases. Controlling your carbohydrate intake along with moderate exercise are tangible steps to decrease the risk of heart disease in diabetic patients. Type 2 diabetes is preventable through a structured lifestyle change program that promotes weight loss, healthy eating, and increased physical activity such as the National Diabetes Prevention Plan.[19]

Summary

Chronic diseases such as heart disease, high blood pressure, and diabetes are increasing in the US and particularly for individuals in Southern states. Patterns of poor eating habits and physical inactivity have contributed to obesity rates and the onset of chronic diseases in the South. As you age, it is important to live a healthy lifestyle if you are at risk for these diseases.

Although heart disease is not reversible, you can control it with diet and lifestyle changes if diagnosed with it. If you have not been diagnosed with heart disease, there are ways to prevent it. In many cases, high blood pressure and type 2 diabetes are preventable, reversible, and/or controllable. When taking medication, a change in lifestyle may enhance the effectiveness of the medication. Please consult a physician before making any changes to medication. An uncontrolled or undiagnosed chronic disease could cause additional health issues.

Chronic diseases cause death and disability within the US daily. Delay, prevention, or reversal of chronic diseases can happen by diet and lifestyle changes. The first step to changing the outcomes of your health is awareness of your risk factors. This book lists five simple steps to jumpstart your health journey regardless of your current diet and gives suggestions for implementing the steps.

Questions for reflection

1. Does your family have a history of chronic diseases? If so, which one(s)?

2. Do you have chronic disease(s)?

3. Do you have a condition that could lead to a chronic disease?

4. Is your disease(s) reversible through diet and lifestyle changes? Yes or No

5. If yes, what can you do to improve your condition?

6. If no, what can you do in addition to taking medication that will improve the effectiveness of your medication?

7. Have you been diagnosed as pre-diabetic? Yes or No

8. What steps can you take to decrease the risk of becoming diabetic?

9. Has a family member been diagnosed with a chronic disease? Yes or No

10. If yes, how can you support your family member?

2

Goodness Gracious!

Lay Your Burdens Down

If the Son therefore shall make you free, ye shall be free indeed.

—John 8:36

Southern funerals, also referred to as homegoings, are different from those in other parts of the United States. Whether a jazz funeral, a unique wake, or an extravagant ceremony, the event is well planned and organized by the funeral home and the church. Normally, the family of the deceased is dressed in modest black or dark clothing. As a child, southern funerals were long. They lasted at least two or three hours and included condolences from friends, community members, family, and the best soloists in town. Sometimes, funeral-goers shouted, "Take me with you!" or "I will see you in heaven." A full church service follows with the Pastor preaching a sermon with an altar call. On the way to the graveyard, true Southerners pull over to the side of the road until a funeral procession passes them on the road, a sign of respect for the mourners. The bereaved family receives an outpouring of support from the church and community.

In terms of food, it is a Southern tradition to bring food to the bereaved family's home before, during, and after the funeral. But it is also a ritual to show love and ease the burden of the loss. The ladies at church plan the food delivery to a grieving family with elaborate casseroles, cakes, and pies. The bereaved family has food to eat for a week or more. The repast, sometimes referred to elsewhere as the after-funeral-luncheon, is another special event held at the church or local community center after the funeral and the graveside service. The family shares a large meal complete with southern favorites like fried chicken, macaroni and cheese, vegetables, and of course, many decadent desserts. The repast is time for the bereaved family to be surrounded by friends, family, and the community.

Since we are talking about funerals, I would like to address the reasons why you have negative eating emotions and habits so you can lay these feelings and practices to rest. I'll provide scientific and spiritual evidence for negative emotions and habits and how they lead to chronic diseases. I will also provide ways that faith will help you to overcome these negative emotions and habits.

Emotional eating in the South

Most Southerners are emotional eaters. They make sure food is at the forefront of most events, whether it is tea, a cotillion, football party, or a funeral. Some of you have witnessed emotional or stress eating in your families. Many southern foods are high in fat, salt, and sugar, and can feed stress or emotional cravings. Here is the cycle. When you feel stressed, the chemicals in your brain responsible for happiness naturally decrease. When that happens, you crave unhealthy food high in fat, salt, or sugar. Eating these increases chemical levels, which makes you feel happy. So, you repeat the cycle when you feel stressed again. The cycle is like those addicted to drugs. Sugar has been described as an addictive drug.[1] Food companies capitalize on how you react to stress by eating and thus begins your addiction to certain foods. With these emotions and stress cycles, you overeat and your bodies store fat, which causes you to gain weight to the point of being overweight or obese. Obesity increases your chances for developing chronic diseases.

Body, soul, and spirit

You are composed of three parts: your body—sometimes referred to as flesh, your soul—sometimes referred to as the mind, and your spirit. All three parts are influenced by the others, so they are all equally important when it comes to changing eating habits. Whatever affects your bodies also affects your souls and spirits. Your body is your outside appearance, the shell covering you live in, and it is composed of cells and houses your internal organs. Your soul refers to how you relate to people—your emotions, feelings, and personality. Whether you feel happy, sad, or depressed is all associated with the feeling of your soul. Soul feelings can be conscious or subconscious. Then, there is the spirit. The spirit is what connects us to a higher power. In my case, my spirit is connected to God. If your souls and spirits are troubled or disconnected, it will influence your health, eating habits, and body.

ACE Study

Science agrees with the body, soul, and spirit connection and its effect on eating habits and health outcomes. Unfortunately, negative emotions and habits may have begun in childhood. One study called the Adverse Childhood Experience Study, or ACE study, was conducted and determined that trauma and toxic stress in childhood increases risk for long-term health and behavioral issues.[2] For example, a traumatic childhood event is responsible for the unhealthy habits, negative emotions, and addictions we have as an adult. Examples of a traumatic childhood event or ACEs is as follows:

- Neglect
- Rejection
- Abandonment
- Abuse
- Loss of a parent through divorce or death
- Parent with a mental illness or substance abuse issue
- Rape or assault

Another study related with ACEs further describes the more adverse events one has as a child the more obesity he/she has as an adult.[3] Unresolved issues from the trauma of childhood may have caused obesity, and obesity increases the risk for chronic diseases.

Spiritual roots of diseases

The ACE study provides scientific evidence linking childhood trauma to obesity. It also shows the body, soul, and spirit connection. Let's look deeper at the spiritual roots or origins and negative emotions associated with chronic diseases. Dr. Henry Wright, who spent twenty years of ministry teaching and researching the spiritual roots of diseases is the author of A More Excellent Way: Be in Health.[4] Dr Wright quoted "80% of all diseases both biological and psychological, is rooted in separation from God, yourself and others." His research aligns with the body, soul, and spirit connection. As was mentioned in Chapter 1 of this book, several diseases are associated with heart disease such as heart attack, hypertension, stroke, and coronary artery disease. Dr. Wright describes the roots of heart disease as a result of fear, anxiety, and stress and explains with a Biblical example. In Luke 21:26 it states, *"Men's hearts fail them for fear and for looking after those things which are coming on earth; for the powers of heaven shall be shaken."* Many people have constant stress and fear over things they cannot change including the things that will come. Recent reviews have also linked ACEs to heart disease in adults.[5]

Wright discusses the spiritual roots of some diseases are:
- Self-bitterness
- Self-rejection
- Self-hatred
- Anger
- Rage
- Resentment

In the case of type 2 diabetes, Dr. Wright describes the root issues as fear—fear of man, fear of failure, and fear of failing others—which relate to an increased number of diabetes cases.

Because physicians focus on your physical bodies, they may not be aware of deep-rooted emotions and feelings you are holding on to because of current issues or issues of the past. All diseases are not caused by spiritual issues or roots; however, many arise due to negative emotions and feelings. These emotions cause your bodies to go to and remain in stress mode, including the hormones related to stress—cortisol and adrenaline—which are released. Even though cortisol is one of the stress hormones, it also regulates blood pressure, increases glucose metabolism, and reduces inflammation. Adrenaline is normally released during the fight-or-flight response required in times of threat. Being stressed and in this mode continuously may cause overproduction of hormones and health issues. It is important to identify the source of your stress. Is the stressful situation temporary? Was an event in the past the cause for your long-term or chronic stress?

Does food provide you with comfort and relief? Is something troubling your soul or spirit that causes you stress or to over-eat and ultimately affects your body?

Before you take physical and medical steps for your health, you need to ask God to reveal to you any unforgiveness, anger, or rage that exists which causes you to have unhealthy eating habits or disease. It is important to seek medical advice and take medication if directed to do so, but it is crucial to examine your negative emotions, behaviors, and eating habits as well. Negative emotions, which may be present in your lives, include guilt, anger, resentment, low self-worth or low self-esteem, self-rejection, or sins such as unforgiveness or bitterness. These emotions cause you to develop unhealthy behaviors or may be the root cause of an existing illness. If you believe in God's word and know that He wants you to have an abundant life but you are dealing with traumatic childhood issues that cause poor health, then you cannot effectively live out your purpose here on earth.

Here is my food story. I did not have a bad relationship with food, but I had a bad relationship with myself caused by some traumatic childhood experiences. I did not value myself enough to think that I deserved to be healthy, happy, or successful, so my negative emotion was self-rejection. Specifically, I dealt with unresolved hurt from childhood and did not focus on my health. As an adult, more hurt and pain occurred, and it caused me to think that it was normal (life is full of ups and downs, after all). So, I suppressed my feelings because I did not know that was abnormal. These actions affected my everyday life, and I did not think my family medical history could change, so there was no need to eat healthy. Instead, I utilized my friendships, prayer, deliverance, and healing from trauma and pain to feel free to love God and myself.

Afterwards, I began to eat healthier foods, my brain fog went away along with anxiety and cravings. Even my dental health improved, and extra weight fell off my body. I think that extra weight was not only an indication of my poor eating habits, but it was also an indication of not getting enough rest and sleep. After you minimize stress, then you can rest easier. Making changes did not happen quickly. It was a process that started by changing my mindset. When my mind changed, my motivation and my actions changed. The same discipline I had with food began to trickle down to other areas in my life such as finances and relationships.

Summary

At Southern funerals, friends, family, and community comforts the bereaved family. Food is again at the forefront of the funeral rituals at home and church. In life, only God can solve, heal, and put issues to rest. Many of you feel stressed and eat foods you think will make you feel better. Unfortunately, after the comforting feeling from the food goes away, the problem remains. As a health coach, I have seen individuals not value themselves because of the guilt, pain, and condemnation they feel from experiences that occurred in their life. The experience could be the death of a loved one, a poor or nonexistent relationship with a parent, a bad relationship, a traumatic event that occurred as a child such as molestation, abuse, a parent's divorce, your divorce, or (insert issue here). These experiences affect all aspects of your life like your mind and spirit and not just your health and body.

Food is meant for enjoyment and to provide nutrition for your bodies. Sadly, poor food traditions, low self-esteem, unforgiveness, and the need for inner healing and trauma are some of the reasons that you have unhealthy eating habits. God's love is unconditional, regardless of what you have experienced in your life. There is nothing you have done or has been done to you that can separate us from Christ's love and His best for you.

This book contains some steps to get you on the right track with healthy eating, but until you surrender your issues to Christ and fully embrace His love, no diet or eating plan will last. You need to ask God to heal the broken and void places in your heart in the same way He did in my life. "*Stand fast therefore in the liberty wherewith Christ hath made us free and be not entangled again with the yoke of bondage*" (Galatians 5:1). For some of you, once you are free to feel His love, you may be able to focus on your health. Now it is time for the death of your trauma which opens the door to a new mind, spirit, and body. First, read and answer the questions below. Next, if you have not accepted Jesus Christ as your Savior, you should do this first. A prayer for this follows the questions below. If you have given your life to Christ, skip to the second prayer. Scriptures for comfort and guidance follow.

Questions for reflection

1. Did you experience trauma as a child or adult?

2. Do you have feelings of low self-esteem or low self-worth?

3. Do you harbor feelings of unforgiveness, anger, rage or rejection, self-rejection, bitterness?

4. What are your sources of stress?

5. Are your stressors things that you can change?

Prayer of Salvation (if you have never accepted Jesus Christ as your Savior)

Please say this prayer if you would like to invite Jesus into your life and you have never accepted Jesus Christ.

Dear Lord Jesus, I admit that I am a sinner. I repent and ask you for forgiveness. I believe that you are the son of God and died on the cross for me to be saved. I receive you in my heart and life as my Lord and Savior. Thank you for hearing my prayer. In Jesus' name. Amen.

Congratulations! If you have prayed this prayer for the first time, you are now saved, and this is the first step in your relationship with Christ. Follow these next steps:

1. Read the Bible
2. Pray
3. Tell others
4. Find a local Bible-based church

Prayer of surrender (if you have accepted Christ)

Lord Jesus, reveal to me the things that happened in my childhood or adulthood that has caused me not to maintain my health. Forgive me for sins and habits that I have participated in because of trauma and forgive me for any destructive and negative behaviors that I have done to worsen my health. Now I know my body, soul, and spirit are connected. Help me to resist temptation from bad food (insert your bad food(s) or issue here). Please bring people around me who offer words of love, support, and encouragement for better health. Show me daily what I need to do to improve my health and lifestyle so I can fulfill my purpose on earth. Thank you, Jesus, for inner healing and your unyielding love and support of me.

Thank you, Jesus, for your power and unconditional love. In Jesus' name. Amen.

Here are some scriptures for comfort and guidance.

Meditate on these scriptures.

Isaiah 43:18-19. *"Remember ye not the former things, neither consider the things of old. Behold I will do a new thing; now it shall spring forth; shall ye not know it? I will make a way in the wilderness and rivers in the desert."*

Romans 12:2. *"And be not conformed to this world; but be ye transformed by the renewing of your mind, that ye may prove what is that good, and acceptable, and perfect will of God."*

1 Corinthians 10:13. *"There hath no temptation taken you but such as is common to man: but God is faithful, who will not suffer you to be tempted above that ye are able; but will with temptation also make a way to escape, that ye may be able to bear it."*

Psalm 32:7. *"Thou art my hiding place; thou shall preserve me from trouble; thou shall compass me about with songs of deliverance. Selah."*

Psalm 34:4. *"I sought the LORD, and he heard me, and delivered me from all my fears."*

Psalm 34:17. *"The righteous cry, and the LORD heareth, and delivereth them out of all of their troubles."*

1 Peter 5:8-9. *"Be sober, be vigilant; because your adversary the devil, as a roaring lion, walketh about like a roaring lion seeking whom he may devour. Whom resist stedfast in the faith, knowing that the same afflictions are accomplished in your brethren that are in the world."*

3

Makin' Groceries

Step 1: Read Your Labels

The heart of the prudent getteth knowledge; and the ear of the wise seeketh knowledge.

—Proverbs 18:15

The first time I heard a friend from New Orleans say, "making groceries," I thought that she was literally going to produce the groceries. She explained the saying "making groceries" comes from the French term "faire son marche" which means "to do one's market shopping." Food traditions in Louisiana, such as crawfish etouffee, red beans and rice, and gumbo and po' boys are different from the delicacies cooked in my small town in Alabama, but the common theme was the food was made with love and from scratch. All sauces and soups were made from scratch, nothing from a jar or can. Fresh greens, vegetables, seafood, and meat were all purchased from local farmer's markets. As we became older, there were more foods available in bags, boxes, and cans that made cooking faster and more convenient. Although there were more food choices for the cooks in our families, the food never tasted the same as when we were younger. Were we getting the same nutrients as when we consume food made with the fresh ingredients? Today, many of you use packaged or processed foods in your daily meals, and it is important to read the nutrition facts label to make sure you know what is in the foods you cook and eat.

In this chapter, we will discuss how to read the nutrition facts label and the ingredients list. This chapter is an important one because if you do not know what is going into your bodies, you will not know how to make better food choices.

Being a wise shopper

Proverbs is one of the books in the Bible in the Old Testament that talks about wisdom, understanding, and fearing God. Proverbs 18:15 states, "*The heart of the prudent getteth knowledge, and the ear of the wise seeketh knowledge.*" The first part of the verse says the heart of the prudent getteth knowledge. The word *prudent* means acting with or showing care for the future. Changing your diet and lifestyle to live a better life is a way you show you have a prudent heart and will find the information you need. The second part of the verse means that you are teachable and looking for evidence to maintain your health. Reading nutrition facts labels is one way to show you are prudent. Let us now discuss the nutrition facts label.

What is the nutrition facts label?

The nutrition facts label is the label on the food that has the number of calories and specific nutrients contained in a food item. The U.S. Food and Drug Administration (FDA) requires packaged foods in the US have food labels. Raw fruits, vegetables, and some fish do not have nutrition labels.

Some coffees and teas and other items like food color contain insignificant amounts of nutrients and do not have to be labeled. Nutrients are any substances that provide nourishment. Your bodies need some nutrients more than others. By reading the nutrition facts label, you will also know what foods to avoid if you have health conditions or are on a special diet. Knowing what goes into your body is powerful, you choose what goes in and how much.

In 2016, the FDA changed the original nutrition facts labels because researchers realized the link between diet, obesity, and chronic diseases. The new changes will help you make better food choices. All labels will be changed by July of 2021.[1] Some manufacturers have not yet switched to the new nutrition facts labels. I will discuss the original nutrition facts labels and the changes to the new labels throughout the following section. The same general rules apply for determining whether a food is healthy or not with both the original and new nutrition facts labels.

The following chart is for reference only and it depicts the original nutrition facts label compared to the new label. [2] According to the FDA, the images above are intended for illustrative purposes only. They are hypothetical labels and represent two fictional products.

Nutrition Facts

Serving Size 2/3 cup (55g)
Servings Per Container About 8

Amount Per Serving

Calories 230　　　　　Calories from Fat 72

　　　　　　　　　　　　　　　% **Daily Value***

Total Fat 8g	**12%**
Saturated Fat 1g	**5%**
Trans Fat 0g	
Cholesterol 0mg	**0%**
Sodium 160mg	**7%**
Total Carbohydrate 37g	**12%**
Dietary Fiber 4g	**16%**
Sugars 12g	
Protein 3g	

Vitamin A	10%
Vitamin C	8%
Calcium	20%
Iron	45%

* Percent Daily Values are based on a 2,000 calorie diet. Your daily value may be higher or lower depending on your calorie needs.

	Calories:	2,000	2,500
Total Fat	Less than	65g	80g
Sat Fat	Less than	20g	25g
Cholesterol	Less than	300mg	300mg
Sodium	Less than	2,400mg	2,400mg
Total Carbohydrate		300g	375g
Dietary Fiber		25g	30g

Nutrition Facts

8 servings per container
Serving size　　　　**2/3 cup (55g)**

Amount per serving

Calories　　　230

　　　　　　　　　　　　　% **Daily Value***

Total Fat 8g	**10%**
Saturated Fat 1g	**5%**
Trans Fat 0g	
Cholesterol 0mg	**0%**
Sodium 160mg	**7%**
Total Carbohydrate 37g	**13%**
Dietary Fiber 4g	**14%**
Total Sugars 12g	
Includes 10g Added Sugars	**20%**
Protein 3g	

Vitamin D 2mcg	10%
Calcium 260mg	20%
Iron 8mg	45%
Potassium 235mg	6%

* The % Daily Value (DV) tells you how much a nutrient in a serving of food contributes to a daily diet. 2,000 calories a day is used for general nutrition advice.

Similarities and Differences in the Original and New Nutrition Facts Label

Original Label	New Label
Daily values	Updated daily values
Calories section	Larger font for the calories section
Contains the serving size at the top of the label	Serving sizes have larger, bolder font and updated for certain foods
Total fat, saturated fat, and trans fat amounts	No change
Cholesterol amount	No change
Sodium amount	No change
Total carbohydrate, dietary fiber, and sugars	Same information with total sugar and added sugars' amounts
Protein is listed	Protein is listed
Percent daily value only contains percentages	Actual amounts of percent daily value on label for vitamins and minerals
Contains vitamins A, C, calcium, and iron	Change in nutrients required; potassium added to labels; Vitamin D added, vitamins C and A removed.
Percent Daily Value based on 2,000 and 2,500 calories	New footnote about percent daily value and only for 2000 calories

I am sure there are plenty of questions. What does all this mean? What do I need to look for on the nutrition facts label? Why does this matter? Let us begin with the serving size and move through the label.

The Serving Size

You should first look at the serving size located at the top of the nutrition facts label. The serving size is in a unit such as pieces, slices, or cups. If the serving size is one cup and you eat the entire package, which is two cups, you must multiply all the nutrients (calories, sodium, and sugar, etc.) on the label by two. On the other hand, if the amount per one serving of a soft drink is twenty ounces—one bottle—and you drink half of the bottle, then you divide the nutrition facts on the label by two. The serving size is one of the most important sections on the label. By looking at the serving size, you can determine how much of a food to eat and what nutrients are included in how much you eat.

Calories

The next section is the calorie section. I do not count calories with my clients because each one of them has a different amount of physical activity. But since I frequently get this question, consuming 2000 calories per day in your daily diet is a standard amount in most meal plans. This means everything you eat in a day equals 2000 calories. It is important to talk with your nutritionist or dietician to determine how many calories you need per day. Typically to lose weight, you must burn more calories than you consume. My general advice is to make calories count by eating nutritious foods. In other words, do not eat something unhealthy that consumes your calories. For example, if the two options are a healthy piece of fruit or an unhealthy cookie, eat the fruit. The piece of fruit will most likely contain more fiber and healthy sugar, while a cookie may contain artificial sugars and no fiber. Regularly consuming large amounts of calories could lead to being overweight or obese.

How much is too many calories in a food?

If the food item contains 400 or more calories for one serving, it is a high calorie food. If possible, you should select a lower calorie food choice. Remember to check the serving size and number of calories per serving. If an item contains two servings in a package and the number of calories per one serving is 400, then consuming the entire package is 800 calories.

Calorie Guidelines for One Food Serving- Based on a 2000 Calorie a Day Diet
400 or more calories are high
100 calories are moderate
40 or less calories are low

Percent (%) Daily Value (DV)

The percent daily value is found on the right side of the label and tells you how the nutrients in one serving of food contribute to your total daily diet. The value is based on a 2000-calorie diet and can be used to select foods that are healthier. If a food has 5% of the %DV or less in a nutrient, it is low in that nutrient. 20% or more of the %DV is high in the nutrient. Use the %DV to compare foods that have nutrients that you need to eat healthier. Let's call it the 5/20 rule. Your goal is to keep the %DV at 5% or lower on nutrients you want to limit (i.e. fats, cholesterol, and sodium), and try to increase your %DV on nutrients that your body needs (i.e. calcium, iron, potassium) to 20% or higher. Please note that *trans* fat, protein, and sugar do not have %DV on the nutrition facts label.

Let's look at the total fat, cholesterol, and sodium sections on the food label. In these sections, there are no changes on the new label.

Total Fat

The total fat section is made up of saturated fat and *trans* fat. You want to limit foods with these nutrients. Eating too many of these nutrients increases your risk of chronic diseases like diabetes, high blood pressure, or heart disease. Total fat indicates how much fat is in the food item. It is broken down into saturated fat and *trans* fat.

Saturated fat

Saturated fat raises your level of cholesterol in your body and is found in red meats, cheese, whole milk, and some baked goods and fried foods. Foods high in saturated fats are also high in calories. You can eat thirteen grams of saturated fat per day or 120 calories in a 2000 calorie diet.

Trans fats

Some *trans* fats occur naturally in animals, and others are produced industrially by adding hydrogen to oils to make them more solid. These fats also increase your LDL or bad cholesterol level and should be limited to 5%-6% of your total calories. They are found in unhealthy foods like doughnuts, baked goods, pie crusts, biscuits, frozen pizza, cookies, and crackers. In the ingredients list of foods, they are listed as "partially hydrogenated oils." We will discuss the ingredients list later in this chapter.

Cholesterol

Cholesterol is found in shrimp, egg yolks, whole milk, and organ meats. It is necessary for production of bile, a fluid made by the liver that aids in digestion of fat. You need less than 300 mg per day. You need to keep these items as low as possible each day to help reduce the risk of diseases. You do this by looking at a variety of foods and consuming the ones with the lowest amounts.

Sodium

Sodium is responsible for vital functions in the body. Too little or too much sodium is bad for your body. According to the 2015-2020 Dietary Guidelines for Americans, individuals need to consume less than 2300 mg sodium or the equivalent of one teaspoon of salt per day.[3] Individuals who have high blood pressure need to consume lower amounts of sodium, as physicians recommend. Athletes or participants in rigorous exercise may need to consume more sodium (check with your nutritionist). Excess sodium is not ideal for the body and increases the risk of chronic diseases. When reading labels, you need to be able to choose lower sodium foods. For sodium, if the %DV of sodium in a food is 20% or more, it is a high sodium food. If the food has a %DV of 5%, it is a low sodium food. Please refer to Chapter 4 in this book for more information about sodium and how to lower your daily intake.

Total Carbohydrate

On the original label, total carbohydrate is subdivided into dietary fiber and sugar. On the new food label, total carbohydrates are broken into dietary fiber, total sugars, and added sugar. Carbohydrates are the main source of the body's energy. Carbohydrates make up 45-65% of our daily caloric intake. The same rules apply for food items and %DV. 5%DV means a food is low in this nutrient, and 20% or greater means the food has a high amount.

Dietary fiber is in the carbohydrate section of the original and new label. Dietary fiber is a type of carbohydrate the body cannot break down, and it passes through the body undigested. Dietary fiber is important for digestion. The DV for dietary fiber is twenty-five to thirty-five grams, so you want to eat high fiber foods. For adult women up to age fifty, the recommended intake is twenty-five grams and men thirty-eight grams. For adult women over fifty, dietary fiber intake should be twenty-one grams and for men, it should be thirty grams daily.[4] Please read more information about the importance of fiber in Chapter 7 in this book.

Sugars are important for energy, but many foods contain added sugars. These sugars are added to the foods and beverages when they are processed or prepared. You need to limit the amount of added sugars in your diet. The AHA recommends that women limit added sugar to six teaspoons or twenty-five (25) grams per day, while men should stick to nine teaspoons or thirty-six (36) grams.[5] Too much sugar has been linked to obesity, and chronic disease.[6] The new nutrition facts labels include added sugar but foods with the old labels do not, so it is important to know the names of added sugar in your foods.[7] Refer to Chapter 5 to read more about sugars, their names, and how to reduce your daily intake.

Vitamins and minerals

These nutrients are important to keep your body functioning properly, so it is important to check %DV of the following nutrients. Twenty percent (20%) DV of a vitamin or mineral is a good amount for your daily total, while 5%DV is a small amount. Your goal is to get as close to the 100%DV as you can of these nutrients in your foods.

Vitamins and Minerals on the Nutrition Facts Labels

Vitamin or Mineral	Functions in the body	Original or New or Both Labels
Vitamin A	important for a strong immune system, good vision, and cell growth	Original
Vitamin C	important in the repair of tissues and absorption of iron	Original
Vitamin D	important for maintaining strong bones and helps the body to absorb calcium	New
Calcium	important for building strong bones and teeth, blood clotting, and muscle contraction	Both
Iron	needed for hemo-globin, a substance in red blood cells that carries oxy-gen throughout the body	Both
Potassium	key mineral in the body that helps to regulate fluid balance, muscle contractions, and nerve signals in our body	Both

Clean eating vs. ultraprocessed foods

Before I discuss the ingredients list, I want to discuss clean eating. What is *clean eating?* Clean eating describes eating real or whole foods such as fruits, vegetables, whole grains, and minimally processed foods. Processing of foods means that the food has undergone a change before it is sold. Foods can be unprocessed, minimally processed, or ultraprocessed. Unprocessed foods are fruits and vegetables in their natural state. Examples of minimally processed foods are bagged spinach or greens and frozen vegetables with no seasoning or sauce added. Moderately processed foods have more processing such as pre-cooking and mixing before packaging. Examples include pasta and canned vegetables. Heavily processed foods have nutrients and natural colors removed and are full of artificial flavors, dyes, sodium, and sugar, then preservatives are added. Ultraprocessed foods contain many ingredients, require little preparation, and are ready-to eat. Examples include frozen pizza and microwaveable dinners, some packaged sweets, salty snacks, and sugar sweetened beverages. Some processed foods overstimulate your taste buds by adding a great deal of sodium or sugar. These foods may be addictive because of the taste. Over time, minimally processed foods taste bland or boring. Whole foods may be minimally processed like a bag of French fries. For example, the whole food is the potato, so frozen French fries with only a few ingredients are minimally processed food. Whole potatoes in a can are moderately processed. Potato chips with added flavoring and color are ultraprocessed foods. It is important to limit ultraprocessed foods.

You need to eat to nourish your body. This includes your snacks. The way you can determine whether a packaged food is clean or not is to read the product label and ingredients.

Product label and ingredients list

The ingredients on a product label are listed in order of pre-dominance, which means that the ingredient with the highest percentage is listed first. If sugar is the first ingredient on the list, you may not want to eat this food because it means more sugar is in the product than other ingredients. The ingredients list contains ingredients from the eight major allergenic foods—milk, eggs, fish, shellfish, tree nuts, peanuts, wheat, and soy.

Be sure to check for hidden sugars in the ingredients such as high fructose corn syrup. I would avoid all foods that have this ingredient. It may seem difficult at first to find foods that do not contain this ingredient, but with reading more labels, you find brands of food items that do not contain this additive. High fructose corn syrup is a sweetener made from corn starch. Eating too much of this sweetener has been linked to weight gain, type 2 diabetes, and high blood pressure.[8,9]

Artificial food dyes are prevalent in food and drinks we consume in America. These dyes have no nutritional value or health benefit. Additionally, some dyes have been banned in countries in Europe due to the link to behavioral issues in children. Common food dyes are Yellow 5, Yellow 6, and Red 40 which make up 90% of the dyes used in food in America.[10] Our family tries to avoid purchasing foods and drinks that contain artificial dyes. The only surefire way to avoid these dyes is to read the ingredients.

Greenwashing on product labels

Greenwashing is the practice of making misleading claims about the benefits of a product. Many companies try to deceive you by making claims about foods such as low-fat or whole grains or no sugar added. If you read the labels and can decipher some of the code words, you will not be fooled.

For example, many low-fat foods are low in fat but are high in sugar. Many products that claim there is no sugar added contain artificial sweeteners such as sucralose, aspartame, or acesulfame potassium.

You can find healthier foods in all stores, not only in specialty stores. My mother-in-law shopped at a local grocery store and purchased some strawberry preserves. The preserves had five ingredients which I could read and understand. The preserves we regularly consumed contained more than fifteen ingredients including high fructose corn syrup. See Chapter 5 on reducing sugar intake. Reading the ingredients is the only way to know what is in the food you plan to eat.

In most grocery stores, you can find products with many ingredients, and you can find them with fewer ingredients. Just because a food has more ingredients does not mean it is a bad food, but you need to make sure you can read and identify the ingredients. Additionally, if the food is purchased from an expensive store, that does not necessarily mean that the food is healthier. A wise shopper reads the nutrition facts label and product label with ingredients.

Some nutrition and product labels are small and difficult to read. If the nutrition facts label or ingredients list are too hard to see because the labels are too small, please buy a magnifying glass. Yes, I said it—please buy a magnifying glass. When in the grocery store with a magnifying glass and reading a nutrition or product label, if someone asks about the magnifying glass or what you are looking for, you should answer by saying "I am looking for my health." A phone camera also works well for enlarging the labels to see them. You can also quickly look up ingredients using your phone.

Summary

Once you start reading food labels, you cannot panic. You might be surprised at what you have been eating. Making healthier food choices is a journey, so you must be patient and not hard on yourself about what you currently eat. Many of you do not have the option of only cooking from scratch. When you must purchase packaged foods, it is important to buy the healthiest of those foods while you are *making groceries.*

You have completed the first part of the book, *The Awareness Section.* You should now be aware of the Southern eating pattern, chronic diseases that are caused by this pattern of eating, eating habits caused by stress or trauma, recognizing spiritual roots of chronic diseases, and tools to help you read the labels of the food you purchase. Be sure to check out the questions and tips following this section to give more understanding of how this section applies to you. Reading your labels is the first and most important step of the five steps listed in this book. Let us look at the remaining four steps and the second part of the book: Making Better Choices.

Step 1:

Read Your Labels

Questions for reflection

1. Why is it important for you to read food labels?

2. What is a nutrition facts label?

3. What does %DV mean?

4. What nutrients do you need to limit in your diet?

5. What nutrients do you need to eat in high amounts?

6. What is the ingredients list?

7. On the product labels on the ingredients list, what does the first ingredient indicate about the food item?

8. What prevents you from reading the food labels?

9. What two items do you need to look for and avoid in the ingredients list?

Tips for reading labels

Let's apply what you have learned about the nutrient facts label and ingredients on the product label. Before you use your new skills at the grocery store, you should go to your pantry and review the nutrition facts and ingredients of your favorite snack food. You should become familiar with the foods you have in your pantry. Check the serving size. If we are eating more than the serving size, multiply by that number. If you are eating less, divide by that number.

1. Check out the calories per serving. A high caloric food has 400 or more calories.

2. Check sodium, sugar (include added sugar), fiber, potassium, vitamins, and mineral content. Review the %DV and the 5/20 rule.

3. Don't be fooled by greenwashing on labels, low-sugar, low-fat, or no sugar added items. Read the ingredients.

4. Avoid foods with high fructose corn syrup, artificial dyes, and products that contain large numbers of ingredients too hard to pronounce.

PART 2
If the Creek Don't Rise

Making Better Choices

4

Take it With a Grain of Salt

Step 2: Reduce Your Sodium

Let your speech be always with grace, seasoned with salt, that ye may know how ye ought to answer every man.

—Colossians 4:6

Southerners love fried foods. We ate lots of fried food in our home and at the homes of family members. It was not uncommon to see containers with cooked grease on the stoves. The grease was recycled to fry additional food items. We ate fried chicken, hot fried chicken, fried chicken wings, fried okra, fried fish, fried shrimp, fried potatoes, fried green tomatoes, fried pickles, fried turkey, French fries, fried corn, fried pies, fried Oreos, fried peach poppers, fried cheesecake, and hushpuppies. Fried foods have more sodium, saturated fat, and calories. Fried foods contain about 400 or more grams of sodium than if the food item is grilled, broiled, baked, or boiled.

In addition to the fried foods, salt shakers and hot sauce are on the table in Southern homes, ready for use. Family members often reach for the salt shaker before tasting the food, and sprinkle away out of habit.

Highly seasoning foods is commonplace in the South. My daughter went on a middle school field trip to a different city known for not having highly seasoned food. After the students were told they would be served meals during the trip, her classmate jokingly asked her if she would be bringing salt and seasoning in her purse.

Fried foods and those seasoned with lots of salt are delicious but should not be eaten regularly. Sodium brings out the flavor in your foods and is an important mineral in your bodies, but too much sodium is not good for your bodies. We will discuss sodium in scripture, in your bodies, and how to reduce your sodium intake from foods.

Salt, also known as sodium chloride, was used as a preservative during Biblical times because there was no refrigeration. Roman soldiers received salt as an allotment with their wages as a unit of exchange. In Matthew 5:13, salt brought out the flavor in food. Christians are called the salt of the earth. Colossians 4:6 says, *Let your speech be always with grace, seasoned with salt, that ye may know how ye ought to answer every man.* Since salt was valued in Biblical times, our communication should be different and full of positive, kind, and encouraging words. The term "salty" is used to describe the attitude of a person who is angry or upset. Salty is the attitude a person gets when they eat food that is too salty. Too much salt is not good for the food or the body. Let us now explore the role of sodium in your bodies.

Why is sodium important in my body?

Sodium is an electrolyte, a mineral that your body needs in relatively small amounts for body functions. Sodium helps to maintain the balance of other minerals in the fluid in the cells and the blood volume and aids in nerve and muscle function. You *get* sodium through food and drink and *lose* sodium through sweat and urine via your kidneys. Your kidneys are the organs that help to regulate the amount of sodium in the urine. If this balance is disrupted, either too much or little sodium will be in the body. If there is too much sodium (which is normally the case because of the Southern eating pattern), your organs work harder to eliminate the excess sodium. Chronic diseases such as high blood pressure, heart disease, and stroke are directly linked to consuming excess sodium.

Osteoporosis is a disease in which you have low bone mass and loss of bone tissue. This disease causes your bones to become weak and brittle. Too much sodium in your bodies increases the risk of osteoporosis. Excess sodium blocks the absorption of calcium. If you have a low sodium intake, it is easier for calcium to be absorbed, which helps to protect you from osteoporosis.

How much sodium do I need per day?

According to the AHA, you need between 1500 to 2300 mg of sodium per day which is about 0.5 to one teaspoon.[1] Unfortunately, Americans consume between 2900 to 4300 mg, which is about two to 2.5 teaspoons of sodium in daily quantities. If you have elevated blood pressure, reducing your sodium content may help you to not develop high blood pressure. When diagnosed with high blood pressure and prescribed medication, lowering your sodium intake will enhance your response to your medications. Excess sodium has also been linked to other chronic diseases and obesity. Here are more facts about sodium and hidden sources of sodium.

What are hidden sources of sodium?

The problem is not the salt you sprinkle on your food. The problem is many foods that you eat daily. Most sodium in your food does not come from the salt shaker on your table. Only 6% of sodium is added at the table during a meal. Only 5% of sodium is added during the cooking process, and 12% naturally occurs in some foods. Where is most of the sodium from? Most of the sodium that is in your foods come from food processing and restaurant foods.[2]

Reading food labels are important, and sodium is one of the nutrients you want to keep low or less than %DV. Foods can be minimally or highly processed (from Chapter 3 Read your labels). Please begin to read the labels of foods and look for the sodium content. If the food has more than a 20%DV, then rethink eating the food. Highly processed and packaged meals and snacks are some of the foods to avoid. Some examples are processed meats, frozen vegetables prepared in a sauce (even a light sauce), some canned foods, soups, frozen biscuits, frozen pizza, microwave, meals, and packaged salty snacks. Examples of sodium in processed foods are found in the ingredients list as monosodium glutamate, sodium nitrates, sodium phosphates, sodium erythorbate, or sodium ascorbate. These sodium-containing products are found in the total sodium amount listed on the nutrition facts label. Remember to also check the serving size of the food because if the serving size is one-half of a serving, eating the entire package will double the sodium content.

Be aware that some meats are infused with sodium before purchase, such as chicken. This practice, called saltwater plumping, is used to enhance the flavor of the chicken. A few years ago, when our family was eating chicken regularly, I purchased what I thought was healthy chicken, not knowing that it has been infused with sodium to enhance the flavor. It is reported that "sodium levels reach more than 400 milligrams per serving" in some chickens.[3] I prepared the chicken with a sodium-based seasoning, then sometimes I added a sauce that contained even more sodium. We ate the chicken at least twice a week and were not aware the chicken was infused with sodium. It is important to check the poultry food label to make sure it does not contain sodium. If it does, season the poultry with no or low-sodium seasonings.

When eating out, including a fast food restaurant, check the nutrition information of the menu items. This may be time-consuming to do, but it is important to know what goes into your body. One of my favorite lunch restaurants that serves the best fish tacos does not put their nutrition information on their website. Unfortunately, I stopped eating there because I did not know the sodium content of what I was consuming. Many entrees in restaurants contain large amounts of sodium. Sodium is high in fast foods because it enhances the flavor and increases the shelf-life of the foods. Unless you are eating at a high-end restaurant and can tell the chef to prepare a low sodium meal, much of your food is packaged or processed, including salads. If the salad contains meats, cheese, and salad dressing, expect a lot of sodium. Here is an example of the calories and sodium content from a fried chicken salad from a restaurant with cheese and bacon without any salad dressing. The salad has 950 calories and 1460 mg (or about 0.5 a teaspoon) of sodium, which is more than half the sodium a person needs for an entire day. The sodium is in the fried meat, bacon, and cheese. When you add the salad dressing (depending on the type), you add another 300 milligrams of sodium. I have seen restaurant salads with Southwestern or buffalo-flavored meat with all the trimmings, and it contained between 3000-3700 mg of sodium, which is more sodium than you need in a day. Soups are other foods that contain a great deal of sodium. An eight-ounce bowl of chicken tortilla soup or tomato basil soup are delicious on a cold day, but it could contain as much as 1600-2300 mg of sodium, or one-half to one teaspoon. Let's look at the amount of sodium in common fast food items across various restaurants. A medium order of French fries contains about 500 mg of sodium, a cheeseburger 680-798 mg of sodium, fried chicken sandwich between 1400-1600 mg of sodium, five-piece crispy chicken strips between 2000-2300 mg of sodium, and a nine-inch pizza with three meat toppings about 3670 mg of sodium. It is easy to see how the amount of sodium adds up if you eat fast food regularly. Please keep in mind these are examples of fast foods that vary in the amount of sodium, so it is important to read the nutrition facts from the restaurant's website. Some higher priced restaurants may be willing to reduce sodium content or offer a healthier option so be sure to ask.

How do I reduce my sodium intake?

The DASH Diet, also known as the DASH eating plan was developed by experts who realized that we eat too much sodium. The DASH diet stands for Dietary Approaches to Stop Hypertension. This eating plan has been shown to lower blood pressure and LDL or bad cholesterol,[4] the two leading risk factors for heart disease. This eating plan helps to create a heart-healthy eating style for life with no special foods and complete with recipes. The eating plan recommends:
- Consuming less than 2300 mg of sodium per day
- Eating vegetables, fruits, and whole grains
- Eating fat-free or low-fat dairy products, fish, poultry, beans, nuts, and vegetable oils
- Limiting foods that are high in saturated fat, such as fatty meats, full fat dairy products, and tropical oils
- Limiting sugar-sweetened beverages and sweets

Your taste buds get used to high sodium foods, so you crave them. As adults, you serve high sodium foods to your children and grandchildren, and they grow used to the taste of these foods. When lower sodium foods are consumed, they taste *bad,* bland, or just boring to them. As you cook and eat lower sodium foods, your taste buds may go through some changes. Initially, foods may not be as appealing as before. It takes six to eight weeks for your taste buds to get used to eating lower sodium foods, so be patient. Your taste buds will change. Your body will thank you. For more tips to reduce sodium intake, please read the questions and tips after the summary.

Summary

Take it with *a grain of salt* that you eat too much sodium daily. The sodium does not come from the salt shaker but from fried foods, restaurant foods, and processed food from the grocery store. If the food from the grocery store indicates less than 140 mg per serving, it is a low sodium food. If it contains more than 400 mg of sodium per serving, it is a high sodium food, and it may not be the best choice. Also, use the 5/20%DV rule to decipher the sodium content of foods. Remember, these are general rules because each person may have different dietary needs. Sodium brings out the flavor in food, but too much of it makes the food taste bad. Unfortunately, so much of our food contains a great amount of sodium, and our taste buds cannot tell the difference. It is important to use herbs and spices in place of sodium-based seasonings to season your foods. Added sodium has detrimental effects on your bodies and increases your risk of obesity, high blood pressure, and heart disease. It is important to lower your sodium intake for better health. Cooking whole foods at home will help you to monitor how much sodium you are consuming.

Step 2: Reduce Your Sodium

Questions for reflection

1. Is sodium bad for you?

2. Why is it important to reduce your intake of sodium?

3. How much sodium do you need per day? If on high blood pressure medication? If not on high blood pressure medication(s)?

4. What steps will you take to eat less ultraprocessed foods to reduce your intake of sodium?

Tips to reduce sodium

- Remember to check the serving size of the item on the food label.

- Read your nutrition facts label and the ingredients list. Use the %DV 5/20 rule.

- Use herbs and spices to season your food such as rosemary, thyme, bay leaves, basil, garlic, or no-salt spices.

- Purchase no or reduced-sodium food items.

- Limit the use of canned foods.

- Try to eliminate highly processed foods.

- Stay away from frozen vegetables with sauces added.

- Avoid cooking with dried seasoning packets for meals.

- Try to prepare more meals at home.

- Avoid or limit fried foods.

- Avoid fast foods.

- Limit salted butter or margarine.

- Use the DASH diet recipes for lower sodium meals.

5

Gimme Some Suga

Step 3: Reduce Your Sugar

It is not good to eat too much honey: so for men to search their own glory is not glory.

—Proverbs 25:27

We had a small kitchen and because I am the youngest of three daughters, my chores in the kitchen during dinner time were limited. My task was to make the beverages for dinner. On Sunday, the beverage of choice was tea. I had to boil the water and let the tea bags steep for several minutes in the water. We never called the tea *sweet tea*, but it *was* sweet tea. I did not know that there was a beverage called *unsweetened tea*. In our house it was *tea*. It seemed like the main ingredient was the sugar added while the tea was hot, not the water, tea, or lemon slices. *Sweet tea* is a staple in the southern cities some call the "red wine of the South."

A few times per week I made Kool-Aid, which also contained lots of table sugar, water, artificial color, and flavoring.

The Kool-Aid or tea was not made correctly unless it had a certain amount of sugar. I know sweet tea and sugary drinks are southern staples, and I do not want to make life miserable for the sweet tea lovers or the individuals who add sugar to many things they eat and cook. I have known folks to add sugar to pre-sweetened cereals, milk, rice, spaghetti, collard greens, and even grits. Yes, even grits. In my humble opinion, a true Southerner does not add sugar to grits. The sugar we used in our beverages or added to our food items was natural table sugar. Today, drinks and food with excess sugar are processed, pre-packaged, and made readily available to be consumed by Southerners. The accessibility of sugars in your diet coupled with your desire for sweets over time has increased your waistlines and risk for chronic diseases. This leads me to Step 3: Reduce your sugar intake. Before we discuss how to do this, let us talk about sugar.

What is sugar?

Proverbs 25:27 says, *"It is not good to eat much honey."* This portion of the verse refers to Proverbs 25:16 which states, *"Hast thou found honey? Eat so much as is as is sufficient for thee, lest thou be filled therewith and vomit it."* Honey was plentiful and a staple food. Because of its sweetness, we may be tempted to eat a lot of it. Eating too much of it could cause gastrointestinal issues and cause us to vomit. These verses make me think about sugar and the abundance found in our foods today. Whether sugar is natural or added because of its sweetness, we are tempted to eat more of it than we need.

Sugars can occur naturally in foods such as whole fruits and are part of a healthy diet if consumed in the proper amounts. Foods with natural sugars normally contain other nutrients your bodies need. For example, whole fruits like oranges have fiber, potassium, and vitamin C. They are not only nutritious, but the sugars in them take longer to digest, leaving you feeling fuller longer. Additionally, the slow digestion process allows our organs to properly metabolize the sugar. Oranges have been shown to lower your risk for heart disease. Sugars in fruits are naturally occurring and are healthy. It is important to eat fruits regularly because of the natural sugars and health benefits.

On the other hand, added sugars are put in foods during the processing or preparation of them. These sugars are not healthy and are in foods like sweet snack foods and drinks. Foods with added sugars normally are not nutritious but are filled with empty calories. Because your body quickly digests foods with added sugars, your blood sugar quickly spikes, which causes your pancreas to work harder to pump out more insulin. Sugar also increases inflammation in your body, which raises a type of fat in the blood called triglycerides. Eating excess added sugar over time increases weight gain and obesity and the risk of chronic diseases such as type 2 diabetes, heart disease, and stroke.[1]

Growing up, the dentist and your parents told you to eat less candy because excess sugar causes tooth decay and cavities. You remembered this effect of sugar because many of you had dental cavities and had to sit for long hours at the dentist. Other ways that excess sugar affects us is well known. Excess sugar affects your mood. Studies have shown that individuals who have diets high in sugar and processed foods have been linked to increased depression.[2,3] Not only does sugar affect your mood, but it has addictive qualities. When eating sugar, the "feel good" hormone, dopamine is released[4] so your brain wants to repeat that feeling. Some individuals have found it difficult to stop eating sugary foods and have had described symptoms like people who were addicted to illegal substances. I have witnessed individuals who frequently eat sugary foods. Then, when you eat food with less sugar, you say the food is not sweet enough. So, your solution is to go back to eating foods with high amounts of sugar.

High consumption of sugar has also been linked to leptin resistance. Leptin is the hormone that tells you to stop eating. The sugar fructose causes resistance to this hormone, so you may continue to eat even after you are full.[5] This process may aid in weight gain and obesity.

Additionally, skin prematurely ages faster when excess sugar is eaten. Sugars attach to proteins in the bloodstream and form products that damage proteins in the skin.[6,7] Sugar is known to cause inflammation, so foods high in sugar can also cause inflammation which may irritate acne-prone skin.

According to the AHA, the major sources of sugar in the American diet are regular soft drinks, sugars and candy, cakes cookies, pies, fruit drinks (fruitades and fruit punch), dairy desserts and milk products (ice cream, sweetened yogurt, sweetened milk), and other grains (cinnamon toast and honey-nut waffles).[8] Some items you think are healthy are breakfast cereals, granola bars (my weakness), and dried packaged fruit. But sometimes they contain a great deal of added sugar. It is important to read the nutrition facts label and ingredients list.

How much added sugar do I need per day?

The amount of added sugar that a female needs per day is twenty-five grams about 6 teaspoons and 100 calories, and a male adult needs thirty-seven and one half grams or 9 teaspoons per day which is no more than 150 calories.[9] This may not seem like a lot of added sugar, but there are four calories in one gram of added sugar. If the product has twelve grams of sugar/added sugar, then that is forty-eight calories. Americans eat about twenty teaspoons of added sugar per day, which is about two to three times more than the amount we need per day. For example, one twelve ounce can of soda contains 140 calories and thirty-nine grams or about seven teaspoons of sugar. If you drink a soda with every meal, keep in mind that over time these beverages may lead to weight gain.

Let's talk about juices. An eight-ounce glass of orange juice contains about twenty-one grams of natural sugar and is 9% DV of carbohydrates. If the juice is 100% juice and there are no added sugars, then the orange juice could be part of a healthy diet. On the other hand, an eight-ounce bottle of orange punch has forty grams of sugar and thirty-nine grams of added sugars (about 7 teaspoons of added sugar) and is 78% DV of carbohydrates. This is an unhealthy drink. Added sugars add calories but no nutrients. The amount of added sugar or sugar amount combined should be less than 10% of daily caloric intake. The orange juice and orange punch examples reflect choosing natural sugars over added sugars. Individuals who have type 2 diabetes or are at risk for the disease should check with their nutritionist about drinking orange juice because it contains a large amount of natural sugar. Water is always the healthiest drink option.

What are some names for sugar?

If you are going to reduce the amount of added sugars you consume, then you must know what sugars are in your food. There are more than fifty names for sugar. Many processed foods have numerous types of sugars in one product even though the nutrition facts label may indicate a small amount of sugar. The total amount of sugar (grams) may appear to be low on some products but added sugar may be hidden in the ingredients list. Be sure to check the ingredients list for the names of sugar below and where the name is located on the ingredients list. Remember the highest quantity of an ingredient is listed first in the ingredients list, and the lowest amount of an ingredient is listed last.

Names of sugar

agave nectar	fructose
Barbados sugar	glucose
barley malt	golden sugar
barley malt syrup	golden syrup
beet sugar	grape sugar
brown sugar	high fructose corn syrup
buttered syrup	honey
cane juice	invert sugar
cane juice crystals	maltase
cane sugar	maltose
carob sugar	maltodextrin
carob syrup	mannose
castor sugar	maple syrup
coconut palm sugar	molasses
coconut sugar	muscovado
confectioner's sugar	panocha
date sugar	refiner's syrup
dehydrated cane juice	sorbitol
demerara	sorghum syrup
dextrin	stevia
dextrose	treacle
diatase	turbinado sugar
evaporated cane juice	yellow sugar

What is high fructose corn syrup (HFCS)?

High fructose corn syrup (HFCS) is a sweetener derived from corn syrup that was added to foods in place of sucrose in the 1970s. Since this time, HFCS became a replacement sugar because it was cheaper and sweeter, and this sweetener is absorbed quickly by the body. HFCS contains glucose and fructose and is found in many different foods such as energy and sports drinks, fruit juices, breads, breakfast cereals, store-bought baked goods, ketchup, salad dressings, sweet pickles, canned fruit, tomato sauces, frozen pizza, jelly, candy, sweetened yogurt, and ice cream. With so many foods that contain HFCS, it is easy to consume large amounts of it. Some scientists blame HFCS for an increase in appetite, obesity, and the increased risk of chronic diseases, while others compare it to sucrose (table sugar) and report that there are no harmful effects of it.[10,11] Since there are different opinions on whether HFCS is unhealthy or healthy, you should try to avoid all foods that contain HFCS.

What about artificial sugars?

Artificial sugars or sweeteners are man-made sugars that are added to many food products. Some examples include sucralose, aspartame, acesulfame potassium, neotame, and saccharin. Common brand names are Equal, Sweet' N Low, and Splenda. These sweeteners provide no or few calories and no nutrition. Even though some of the artificial sugars are viewed as safe by regulatory agencies, artificial sugars have some contradictory research surrounding them. The American Diabetes Association and AHA have deemed artificial sweeteners useful in helping to reduce calories which may decrease the risk of chronic diseases.[12] Artificial sweeteners are found in some food products such as gum, yogurt, sodas, desserts, and soft drinks. Diet sodas contain artificial sweeteners and have zero sugars and no calories. Some data suggests individuals choose to eat more calories while consuming zero-calorie drinks because they assume they can eat more when calories are not coming from their beverage.

Be leery of products with product labels that read "no sugar added." In most cases, there is an artificial sugar added that is much sweeter than a natural sugar. For example, this label was on a popular sports drink my friend was consuming, so she read the label. She saw sucralose, an artificial sugar, was in the drink. The label was technically correct. Sucralose is not sugar, but it is an artificial sweetener that adds no calories or carbohydrates. It is about 600 times sweeter than natural sugar. Some studies have linked sucralose to health problems if consumed in excess. Other studies claim that sucralose is safe.[12] Since there are mixed views in the scientific arena, I would limit or avoid items containing sucralose. Be careful with "no sugar added" labels or ones that allude to small amounts of sugar. Artificial sweeteners are usually added, so please read the list of ingredients. For diabetics, please consult a doctor about consuming artificial sweeteners.

How do I reduce my sugar intake?

Studies have shown that sugar addiction is real. When you eat sugar, your brain releases dopamine, a feel-good chemical which makes the sugar habit hard to break. It is important not to go cold turkey while giving up sugar. Any substance that mimics addictive substances can be difficult to remove too quickly without some difficulty. Some people experience headaches, stomach aches, or irritability after quickly giving up sugar. It may be best to wean off sugar. It is important to determine how much sugar you consume, which you can figure out by reading nutrition facts labels and the ingredients list on all foods you eat. It is surprising to discover how many foods contain sugar.

Next, I suggest replacing the foods you consume that have added sugars with ones that have natural sugar, like fruits. Also, try to find and eat food products with no added sugars. Be sure to stay clear of products labeled "no sugar added." These products may contain sucralose or other artificial sweeteners. More strategies to reduce sugar intake are below after the questions. As always, before making any drastic changes to a diet, talk to a doctor.

Summary

While I grew up with the table sugar-sweetened sweet tea—not the healthiest choice—it was still a better choice than the sugar-laden drinks available in today's market. Over the past thirty years, sugar has been added to many more food items, which is harmful to your body when eaten in excess. Sugar can be addictive and a difficult habit to break. There are so many negative effects of sugar, and some researchers recommend never consuming added sugars. Whole foods like fruits with natural sugar are the best sources of sugars because they contain other nutrients. Whole fruits like apples do not cause the same surge of feelings that a candy bar would. Eating a donut for breakfast causes a spike in blood sugar and then the usual crash afterward. Better choices are not impossible. Plain oatmeal with fresh berries or plain Greek yogurt and some fresh fruit for breakfast are better choices. They will not cause a blood sugar spike. These choices are healthier and will fill you longer. At first, the food swaps may be boring, but over time, your taste buds will adapt, and your body will thank you. Making healthy choices about sugary foods will nourish your body and avoiding empty calories will not add extra weight.

Step 3:

Reduce Your Sugar

Questions for reflection

1. Why is too much sugar bad for your body? Name two ways.

2. What foods do you consume that contain a large amount of sugar?

3. What are added sugars?

4. How do you find if added sugars are in your food?

5. Are you addicted to sugary foods? If so, what steps will you take to reduce my sugar intake?

Tips to help reduce your sugar

- Make your own trail mix (be sure not to eat it all at one time).

- Each more fresh or frozen fruit.

- Limit or avoid fruit juice.

- Reward yourself with one sugary item each week.

- Drink water instead of juices, -ades, or punch.

- Infuse your water with fruits.

- Buy some carbonated water and add fruit.

- Eat foods with natural sugar (e.g. fruits).

- Make your own tomato sauces.

- Drink unsweetened tea or sweeten the tea with natural sugar.

- Eat plain yogurt with berries.

- Avoid energy drinks and sports drinks (unless you are an athlete).

- Avoid flavored water.

- Avoid sugar-coated cereals and snacks.

- Limit or avoid artificial sweeteners.

6

I am Full as a Tic' on a Dawg

Step 4: Reduce Your Portions

Be not among winebibbers; among riotous eaters of flesh.

—Proverbs 23:20

Eating large portions of food was the norm in many places in the South. We often heard the phrases: "Let that growing child eat!" and "You should eat because you will be hungry later." And "Please get second helpings! Don't be shy eating!" Then, "Take a plate home with you! I will get the aluminum foil." These phrases were typical indicators of Southern hospitality and meant to make the guest feel welcomed and part of the family on holidays, special occasions, or Sunday dinners. Lots of food meant comfort, and the more food I saw, the better I felt. As a child, I knew nothing about food portions. At breakfast as a child, it was not uncommon for me to eat six full size pancakes, bacon, and eggs. At dinner, I ate a full-sized plate of food then a second helping from a large serving dish. The dish was filled to the rim with what I thought was endless food. When we had spaghetti and meat-balls for dinner, I was a happy child. Southern cooks may feel insulted if their guests do not have a second helping. Now, as an adult, I feel that way when I serve people in my home.

I experienced food portion shock as a young adult when I traveled to Washington, DC, to my husband's (my then-fiancé) home for a dinner. His parents both had roots in the South. His father was from Alabama, and his mother's relatives from South Carolina. Therefore, I knew there would be a smorgasbord of food. When we sat down for dinner, I noticed the serving dishes were small and not filled to the rim as they were in my home. I thought, *How is this small amount of food going to be enough for all of us?* I was surprised when we ate and were all *satisfied*, but not full. Before that visit, I thought all families from the South ate lots of food with second helpings. On that day, I realized I was raised in a home and community where we ate large portions of food.

What is a portion? A portion is the amount of food you *choose* to eat for a meal or snack. A portion is different from a serving size, which is a standard amount of food such as an ounce or cup. In Chapter 3, I talked about serving sizes and reading nutrition facts labels. In my Southern culture, there was no limit to the *portion*. There was always plenty, and we ate as much as we wanted and could eat.

As adults, your empty stomachs are the size of a clenched fist and hold about 2.5 ounces. When full, your stomachs can hold about one quart of food and can accommodate by stretching if you overeat. God perfectly designed your bodies. He knew you would not be perfect and would sometimes overeat. The hunger hormone, ghrelin, promotes appetite and tells your brain you are hungry. Leptin, another hormone we discussed in Chapter 5, is produced by fat cells and lets the brain know when you are full. It takes about twenty minutes for your brain to tell your stomach you are full. Therefore, you should eat for a full twenty minutes.

How does it feel when you overeat? You may feel full, stuffed, or bloated. Your stomach protrudes, then you need to unbutton your pants. You might even feel sick like you need to vomit, or you may have heartburn, feel stressed, or sleepy. This is your body's way of telling you, you need to stop eating. Symptoms occur because your organs are working harder to digest food, and more hormones are produced by the endocrine system. Long term overeating may lead to a slower metabolism, weight gain, obesity, and increase your risk for chronic diseases.

Why do you overeat? When I was younger, I thought I was *eating* and didn't realize I was overeating. What I mean is because my family and friends overate, I overate. It was what we did and but for some, it may have been gluttony. Proverbs 23:20-21 states, *"Be not among winebibbers; among riotous eaters of flesh."* These verses describe gluttony and urges us not to hang around people who drink too much wine and eat too much meat. I am aware that not every overweight or obese person practices gluttony. I know some with healthy weight who eat in excess. Gluttony refers to excess in eating or habitual greed. Proverbs 23:2 refers to gluttony as a serious sin. *"And put a knife to thy throat, if thou be a man given to appetite."* Gluttony is not only about eating. It is that you are making the food your God. The implication is if you do not have self-control when eating and drinking, then you may not have control in other areas of your life. Self-discipline is a key factor in growing as a Christian.

Gluttony may not be the reason we overeat in the South; it may be that food is plentiful like at an all-you-can-eat buffet. Growing up in Alabama, I do not remember many buffet-style restaurants, especially not all-you-can eat types, but now they are plentiful. Whether overeating occurs at a restaurant or a family dinner, heavy meals may trigger a heart attack, especially for those with higher risk.

One study with about 2000 people found that people at risk for heart disease were four times more likely to have a heart attack two hours after a big meal. What happens is large, high fat meals can impair the ability of blood vessels to dilate or expand when needed if a person has cardiovascular disease. Eating a large meal causes your heart rate to increase because of the increased demands from the digestive tract. The stress hormone norepinephrine is secreted and can raise blood pressure and heart rate.[1] As you age, your metabolism slows down, and you do not need to force your organs to work harder, so you should eat smaller portions and nutritious food.

Southerners have consumed large portions for generations, but in the last twenty years, restaurant and food industries have not helped the problem. Portions have doubled or even tripled, which leads to more calories (fats, sodium, and sugar) and contribute to the US obesity problem. Even in fast food restaurants, meals are larger even if you do not request it—maybe it would be wiser to purchase a kid's meal. According to the National Heart, Lung, and Blood Institute, here are examples of portion and calorie increases over the last twenty years:

Comparison of Portions and Calories 20 Years Ago to Present Day [2]

	20 Years Ago		Today	
	Portion	Calories	Portion	Calories
Bagel	3" diameter	140	6" diameter	350
Cheeseburger	1	333	1	590
Spaghetti w/meatballs	1 cup sauce 3 small meatballs	500	2 cups sauce 3 large meatballs	1,020
Soda	6.5 ounces	82	20 ounces	250
Blueberry muffin	1.5 ounces	210	5 ounces	500

Meat is for Southerners.

Since we are talking about portion size, our meals in the South were not complete unless half of the plate was filled with meat. We made sure we had a meat with each meal. For Sunday dinner, having two meats like ham and chicken was a special treat. In the South, individuals consume many meats such as rabbit, alligator tail, frog legs, chitlins, hog maws, Rocky Mountain oysters, oxtails, neckbones, sweetbreads, pickled pig feet, slugburgers and chicken gizzards. Many meats were fried with a sauce or high in sodium.

One of my dad's hobbies was deer hunting. The fact of killing an animal and eating it made my sisters and I squeamish. My mother used to prepare venison (deer meat) without us knowing in delicious chilis or stews, and we gobbled them up. Hours after eating, she told us we had eaten *Bambi*, and we would cry.

Is eating meat healthy for you?

The answer to this question depends on who you ask. Perhaps a better question is what *type* of meat is good or bad for you? In 2015, the World Health Organization declared processed meat a carcinogen that increases your risk of colon or rectum cancer.[3] Processed meat includes sausages, hot dogs, bacon, jerky and luncheon meats. So, by these standards, processed meats are bad for you. I recommend you eliminate them from your diet completely or only eat them occasionally. The negatives of eating meat are that meat contains saturated fat and cholesterol. Saturated fat raises your bad cholesterol, or LDL, and is found in red meat, animal-based foods, cheese, and butter. For someone on a 2000 calorie diet, the recommendation is to limit saturated fat to twenty-two grams per day to lower the risk of heart disease.

I want to make you aware of the most comprehensive food study about nutrition conducted over twenty years. It is called the China Study.[4] The study suggests cancer is more often caused by animal proteins than plant-based proteins, and plant-based proteins may improve your health. One of the conclusions in the study indicates that you do not have to eat meat for your recommended nutrients. The article suggests plant-based foods contain all the required nutrients for your health. The study shows that tofu, nuts, and beans are good sources of protein, and plants also contain a great deal of protein. The study also shows that a plant-based diet reduces type 2 diabetes and heart disease as well as certain types of cancer and other major illness. As with many nutrition studies, there is controversy and criticism.

Every time I have given up meat for a fast, I experienced better sleep quality, lost weight, felt lighter, and had more energy. So now, I eat only small amounts of meat per week, if any. I encourage a meatless day at least once a week, which begins by trying a variety of meatless meals. What are some examples of meatless meals? You can make pasta and add veggies instead of meat, or you can make tacos with beans instead of meat. A veggie dinner with no meat includes veggie soup, chili, pizza, or making a veggie burger with chickpeas or other vegetables. If you stop eating meat for long periods of time, you need to be sure you check with your physician or nutritionist to make sure you are getting the proper nutrients, vitamins, and minerals. I am not advocating the reader become a vegetarian, vegan, or pescatarian, but I do encourage you to consume less meat.

For the meat eaters

However, if you prefer to eat meat, then you are getting a high protein source, which contains essential amino acids, vitamins, and minerals. Red meat is a good source of iron and vitamin D for pregnant women and adolescents. Meat keeps you fuller longer, which may aid in weight loss and improves muscle mass in older women.[5] When selecting meats, be sure to consider lean cuts of meat that contain less fat. Examples of healthier meats are sirloin steak, chicken thighs, and pork tenderloin. When preparing meat, you should limit high heat cooking like smoking and charcoal grilling or barbecuing as these ways of cooking meat have been linked to cancer.[6] Be sure to eat smaller portions of meat.

Summary

The Southern tradition is to eat large portions, especially for special occasions. During the Thanksgiving and Christmas holidays, it is easy to gain weight from overeating. As you age, it is important to think about what happens to your digestive system when you overeat. As Christians, you need to exercise discipline in all areas of your life. For some of you, that means decreasing your food portions. Giving up meat once a week is great way to start exercising discipline with food. Since food portions have increased over the years, you need to be mindful of how much you eat. According to the USDA, one way to control portions sizes while cooking at home is to use The Plate Method.[7] The Plate Method asks the consumer to divide the plate into fourths. One-fourth of the plate is meat or another protein source, another other fourth is a starchy vegetable or whole grain, and the entire other half (two-fourths) should have non-starchy or green vegetables.[7] Try this method when eating lunch and dinner. By reducing portion sizes, you can decrease your chances for weight gain, obesity, and developing chronic diseases.

Step 4: Reduce Your Portions

Questions for reflection

1. Do you eat large portion sizes? If so, why?

2. Have you been eating large portions since you were a child? Was it out of habit or tradition?

3. What are you going to do to decrease your portion sizes?

4. Do you eat meat with every meal? If so, why?

5. Are you going to prepare and eat meatless meals once a week?

Tips to help reduce portions

- Stay away from buffets.

- If eating at a restaurant, have your food packaged to go and eat half of it. (Do not do this at a fancy restaurant.)

- Use the plate method for lunch and dinner.

- Eat on a smaller plate.

- Eat foods that require a fork. You consume more food if you eat with your hands.

- Try eating with chopsticks.

- Don't wait until you are famished to eat. Eat smaller meals and healthy snacks throughout the day.

- At dinner, ask for the lunch portion (it may be a smaller portion).

- If eating from a fast-food restaurant, get a kid's meal.

- Skip the appetizers and dessert.

- Make sure you eat healthy snacks between meals. Snacks keep you fuller longer such as fruit and not processed or sugary snacks.

- Drink an eight-ounce glass of water before eating your meal.

7

Snapping Beans, Pickin' Plums, and Shuckin' Corn

Step 5: Eat More Fruits and Vegetables

And God said, Behold I have given you every herb bearing seed, which is upon the face of all the earth, and every tree, in the which is the fruit of tree yielding seed; to you it shall be for meat.

—Genesis 1:29

In the summer, my cousins and I picked bright green plums from my uncle's yard. We shucked vivid yellow corn on the porch that was given to us by a local farmer. My mama grew succulent red tomatoes in her garden. There were always colorful fruits and vegetables around us; an abundance of whole foods with natural color. We ate fruits and vegetables with beautiful red, green, yellow, and purple hues. This was another one of the pleasant things about growing up in the South.

Little did I know, God was color-coding these foods to help our bodies function properly, and He meant for us to eat many of them. Over time, I discovered the colorful foods we ate contained substances called phytochemicals, also known as phytonutrients. "Phyto" means plants, so phytochemicals are substances produced by plants. Phytochemicals not only refer to the colors of the fruits and vegetables but also the texture and the taste. There are thousands of phytochemicals found in fruit and vegetables, but many of them have not been studied widely. Some common ones researched recently are beta-carotene, lycopene, and lutein. These three vitamins, also known as carotenoids, act as fighters (antioxidants) battling against molecules called free radicals which damage our cells. Cell damage from these molecules ultimately causes chronic diseases and cancer.

Phytochemicals are known to reduce the risk of diseases. Research shows a diet high in fruits and vegetables can lower the risk of heart disease, stroke and high blood pressure.[1] The AHA recommends four to five servings each per day, which means four to five servings of fruits and four to five servings of vegetables.[2] One serving of fruit is one medium fruit, *or* ½ cup fresh, frozen, or canned fruit (with no added sugars), *or* ¼ of dried fruit and ½ cup of 100% fruit juice (with no added sugars). You should check with your doctor about your fruit intake if you are a diabetic. For vegetables, one serving is one cup cooked or raw (except for salad greens—two cups equal one serving), *or* a half cup of fresh, frozen, or canned vegetable (use no sodium or reduced sodium brands), *or* a half cup of vegetable juice. More vegetables equal a better boost for your health. Foods with natural colors contain specific nutrients, and each color has a benefit. Let us explore the colors of some fruits and vegetables and their benefits.

Green fruits and vegetables

Green fruits and vegetables have chlorophyll and contain vitamin K, folic acid, and potassium. Green fruits and vegetables are artichokes, asparagus, avocados, bok choy, broccoli, Brussels sprouts, celery, collard greens, cucumbers, green apples, green beans, green cabbage, green grapes, green onions, green peppers, kale, kiwi, leeks, limes, mustard greens, okra, peas, pears, romaine lettuce, snow peas, spinach, sugar snap peas, watercress, and zucchini.

Red and pink fruits and vegetables

Red and pink fruits and vegetables contain antioxidants such as lycopene, found in tomatoes, which are associated with decreased risk of cancer, heart disease, and certain eye disorders. Red and pink fruits and vegetables include beets, cherries, cranberries, pink grapefruit, pomegranates, radicchio, radishes, raspberries, red apples, red grapes, red peppers, red leaf lettuce, red bell peppers, red potatoes, rhubarb, strawberries, tomatoes, and watermelon.

Yellow and orange fruits and vegetables

Yellow and orange fruits and vegetables have beta-carotene and contain vitamin A, which is associated with good vision. Ever heard that you should eat carrots for excellent eyesight? Other yellow and orange fruits and vegetables are acorn or butternut squash, apricots, cantaloupe, corn, grapefruit, lemons, mangoes, nectarines, oranges, orange juice, orange peppers, papaya, peaches, pineapple, pumpkin, summer squash, sweet potatoes, tangerines, yams, yellow apples, yellow peppers, and yellow squash.

Blue and purple fruits and vegetables

Blue and purple fruits and vegetables have a healthy dose of vitamin C, potassium, and folate. More phytochemicals are in darker foods such as blueberries, blackberries, eggplant, currants, dates, purple grapes, plums, prunes, purple figs, and raisins.

White fruits and vegetables

Our final category which you might not consider as colorful is the white fruit and vegetable category. White fruits and vegetables are also important and are high in dietary fiber. White foods are bananas, cauliflower, garlic, Jerusalem artichoke, mushrooms, onion, potatoes, parsnips, and shallots.

Fiber in fruits and vegetables

Growing up in Alabama, when someone became ill with a cold, respiratory illness, stomachache, headache, or almost any other ailment, Southern mamas asked you a series of two questions. They asked about your regularity or candidly when was the last time you had a bowel movement? As embarrassing as this was as a child, I realized that these questions, although rather intrusive, were valid. If your answer was not *the correct one*, the Southern mamas gave you household dose of castor oil (I do not recommend this) to assist in the process. Your food intake and lifestyle habits coupled with aging can contribute to constipation. Fiber helps to get things moving in your systems. As you increase the colorful fruits and vegetables on your plate, we will most likely increase your intake of dietary fiber. Fiber is your friend. As you age, your digestive system may start to slow down, so it is important for you to increase your fiber intake. Fiber makes you feel fuller longer, and fiber keeps everything moving through your digestive tract.

How much fiber do I need each day?

A man fifty years or younger needs thirty-eight grams per day. Women of the same age need twenty-five grams per day. If you are fifty and older, you need thirty grams for a man and twenty-one grams for a woman.[3] Refer back to Chapter 3 about reading labels, nutrition facts, and ingredients to calculate the amount of fiber you consume daily from some packaged foods. Most of you do not get enough fiber in your diets. Because of this, you may experience constipation or bloating. Another possible short-term effect of not having enough fiber is you continue to eat immediately after you finish a meal because remember, foods with fiber keep you fuller longer.

Why do I want to increase my fiber intake?

Fiber aids in passing eliminated waste, relieving constipation, and helping you feel full, which can also help to manage a healthy weight. Fiber, what mama may call *roughage*, helps move substances through your digestive system. Some fruit and vegetables, which contain a higher amount of fiber, are broccoli, cauliflower, green beans, apples, and potatoes. Other food sources with fiber are whole grains, wheat bran, nuts, and seeds. One study in the Lancet found that people who ate twenty-five to twenty-nine grams of fiber per day saw a 15% to 30% decrease in their risk of developing risk of heart disease, diabetes, and colon cancer.[4]

Water in fruits and veggies

In the South, when we were children and played outside with our friends, we were not allowed to frequently come back and forth in the house. We were told that we would be letting the *good* air out of the house. So, we ate honeysuckles or caught lightning bugs (fireflies) in jars. When we were thirsty, we drank from the water hose. Yes, the long tube attached to the side of the house that was used to water the grass, wash the car, and the dogs. We passed the water hose from person to person. I am not sure how sanitary that was, but we were not thirsty after drinking from the water hose. While we were outside playing, there was only water, no sweet tea or Kool-Aid. Nothing quenches thirst on a hot summer day like water from a water hose.

Your water consumption increases when you eat fruits and vegetables, which is beneficial. About 20% of your water intake comes from food. Fruits such as watermelon, tomatoes, and vegetables such as broccoli, cucumber, and iceberg lettuce contain 90% of higher water content (by weight). Many fruits such as strawberries, cantaloupe, grapefruit, peaches, pineapple, plums, and oranges have a large amount of water.

Since we are on the topic of water, it is important to stay hydrated by eating lots of fruits and vegetables but also by drinking plenty of water. Your bodies are made up of 60% water. Water helps to provide the balance of body fluids. Water loss in your body occurs through sweat, urine, stool, breathing, and evaporation. Dehydration occurs when the amount of water you consume does not equal the water leaving your body. Electrolytes such as potassium and sodium can get off balance when you are dehydrated. The kidneys may not be able to function properly since they keep the level of electrolytes stable in the body. Dehydration can also affect the brain and spinal cord. Though you experience the sensation of thirst, sometimes you need water even if you don't feel thirsty. This is especially true when you reach fifty plus years of age. Please drink water even when you are *not* thirsty.

In the South, if you had a headache, felt sluggish, or wanted a snack, mama said, "Go drink some water!" I think they were accurate in their response because sometimes you may have been slightly dehydrated, but your mind told you, you were hungry. So, it is important to drink enough water.

Why is drinking water important?

Here are a few reasons to drink plenty of water:
- Lubricates the joint cartilage
- Improves athletic performance
- Helps the digestive system to flush waste
- Aids in maintaining blood pressure and blood circulation
- Helps with brain function
- Improves focus
- Curbs your appetite and may help with weight loss
- Creates saliva and mucus and reduces tooth decay
- Prevents dry skin

How much water is enough water?

Experts say to drink half of your body weight in water. For example, for someone 150 pounds, you should drink seventy-five ounces of water per day. I like this strategy, but I think it is more important to begin simply by drinking *more* water. If you increase your water intake immediately, you might run to the restroom all day, which could frustrate you and your intent to change your lifestyle. It is better to start with smaller changes. Additionally, when you have an active lifestyle, you may need to drink more water than the equivalent of half of your weight.

How do I know if I am hydrated?

When hydrated, your urine color should be light yellow. If your urine is clear, you might be overhydrated. Please note vitamins, medication, and food can influence urine color.

Summary

The next time you eat a meal, you should look at your plate and see what natural colors are present. If there are not many colors, you should strive to eat more colors for at least one meal. After adding a few new fruits and veggies to one meal, you can eat the natural rainbow by filling your plate with colorful fruits and vegetables at as many meals as you can. When you increase your colors with fruits and vegetables, you can increase your fiber and water intake, which help to boost your health. For example, eating watermelon, which contains more than 90% water and 6-8% natural sugar, has the essential electrolytes of calcium, magnesium, potassium, and sodium along with vitamin C, beta-carotene, and lycopene, which will give the body UV protection. It seems to be an almost perfect and healthy fruit.

God color-coded fruits and vegetables to reduce the risk of diseases and cancers. He knew what He was doing when He made these plants. There are many others colorful fruits and vegetables to try. There are burgundy heirloom tomatoes, Japanese purple sweet potatoes, purple cauliflower, light brown beets, over 160 varieties of green beans, more than fourteen types of lettuce, and 100 varieties of apples commercially grown in the US. Why not treat yourself to some of these colorful and healthy foods? Mama knew what she was talking about when she said eat *all* your fruits and veggies!

Step 5: Eat More Fruits and Vegetables

Questions for reflection

1. How many fruits and vegetables do you eat per day?

2. Do you need to increase the number of fruits and vegetables per day?

3. Why is it hard for you to eat fruits?

4. Why is it hard for you to eat vegetables?

5. How do you plan to eat more fruits and vegetables?

Tips to eat more fruits and vegetables

- Try to eat fruits or vegetables for all meals.
- Hide vegetables in your casseroles.
- Hide vegetables in your sauces.
- Hide vegetables in your smoothies.
- Eat fruits for most of your snacks.
- Always keep fruit with you.
- Try new fruits and vegetables each month.
- Eat fruits and vegetables that are in season (they are less expensive).
- Use the plate method (from Chapter 6, Step 4 Reduce Your Portions).
- Make your own smoothies.
- Eat more salads.
- Make homemade vegetable soups.
- If you are diabetic or pre-diabetic, check with your physician about the amount and types of fruits to consume.

View Appendix A for the dirtiest fruits and vegetables you purchase. If possible, buy the organic varieties of these foods.

View Appendix B for the fifteen fruits and vegetables least likely to contain a pesticide residue. You can purchase these as non-organic or traditional products.

View Appendix C, it gives information on whether a fruit or vegetable is organic.

PART 3

Who are your people?

Accountability Is the Key to Success

8

I Am Sweatin' Like a Sinner in Church

Exercise and Sleep

I beseech you therefore brethren, by the mercies of God that ye present your bodies a living sacrifice, holy, acceptable unto God, which is your reasonable service.

—*Romans 12:1*

Growing up in Alabama, we thrived on outside activities. My sisters, neighbors, cousins, and I stayed active daily by playing kickball, baseball, cycling, or simply walking to the corner store. Walking to and from school or walking with cousins to and from the local public library were all normal activities. At the library, we picked ten books each, which we planned to read within two weeks. It is odd we never had a bag or box to carry these books.

Not only did the children get plenty of exercise, but the adults did too by gardening, washing cars, raking leaves (when the children didn't have to do it), and chopping wood, which we had to carry to different locations. Saturdays we cleaned and danced to the R&B songs played on the large floor model stereo. This was a common practice in many Southern families.

Even when my sisters and I went to the Midwest to spend summers with my grandmother, we walked her dogs in the nearby park or hopped on or off city buses to run errands with her. Over the last twenty years, society has become more sedentary. We sit in front of a computer or couch and watch TV. We play on our mobile phones or video games for hours without moving. We only get up to get a snack and to go the bathroom. These inactive ways along with poor eating habits have increased our risk for chronic diseases.

I have provided five simple steps to jumpstart your health journey:

1) Read your labels.
2) Reduce your sodium.
3) Reduce your sugar.
4) Reduce your portions.
5) Eat more fruits and vegetables.

There are so many more tips and steps to improve your health such as scheduling annual medical appointments and reducing stress. In my health coaching practice, I focus on foods and eating habits, which I think is 80% of the battle, but exercise and sleep are the other keys to the puzzle of maintaining health.

In the past year, I have attended birthday parties of a ninety-year-old, eighty-year-old, and seventy-five-year old friends. What they all had in common was they had no health issues, and they all exercised daily. Their exercise routines were not the same, but they all kept their bodies moving like we did growing up in the South. The ninety-year-old walked every day for at least thirty minutes. The eighty-year-old worked in her garden and took line dancing classes. The seventy-five-year-old went to the local YMCA, swam, and lifted light weights. For these seniors and you, exercise is the magic pill. God designed your bodies to move. There are countless reasons why exercise is beneficial for your bodies and health. Here are a few reasons why consistent exercise is so important.

Exercise improves mood. In a previous job, I had a difficult work environment, and I started to walk for thirty minutes before my lunch break. When I returned from the walk, I felt revived and happy. Exercise improves your mood by the stimulating brain chemicals like serotonin that make you feel happy and relaxed. Genetic research also shows that exercise can protect against the risk of depression[1] and regular moderate exercise reduces depression and anxiety.[2]

More benefits of exercise include improved muscle strength, increased endurance, and more energy. Your muscles get stronger the more you use them. Some exercises build muscles, which makes them more able to support your joints. As you age, it is important to exercise for living or functional fitness. Functional fitness is being able to bend and stretch to do everyday things such as getting groceries out of the car, climbing stairs, or bending down to pick up items with ease. Balance and coordination are needed to perform these activities. So, it is important to implement exercises to increase muscle strength.

Furthermore, your aerobic capacity increases with consistent exercise and increases in endurance. While exercising, oxygen and nutrients are delivered to your cells, and your aerobic capacity increases. This occurs when you walk up the same flight of steps over time. Eventually, walking up the flight of steps is not difficult, and the length of time it takes decreases.

Most importantly, exercise can help to prevent or manage chronic diseases such as high blood pressure and type 2 diabetes. Weight loss also occurs through daily physical activity. Regular exercise causes your body composition to decrease, which reduces the risk of developing some diseases.

We have discussed some of the benefits of exercise. Here are some guidelines for adults and exercise. Keep in mind these are only guidelines. You should find an exercise you enjoy and consult your physician when you start any exercise program.

According to the Department of Health and Human Services, the Physical Activity Guidelines for Americans provides a comprehensive set of recommendations for Americans on the amounts and types of physical activity needed each day. Adults aged eighteen to sixty-five need at least 150–300 minutes of moderate aerobic exercise each week. This is equivalent to seventy-five to 150 minutes of vigorous-intensity aerobic physical activity, which is also equivalent to a combination of moderate and vigorous intensity aerobic activity. Adults should also do muscle-strengthening activities two or more days a week. Adults older than sixty-five should do a multicomponent physical activity that includes balance training as well as aerobic and muscle strengthening activities. If you have a chronic condition or disability, if able, you should follow the previous guidelines for adults and do both aerobic and muscle-strengthening activities.[3]

One suggestion for the aerobic activity is thirty minutes of a moderate paced walk on most days of the week. Additionally, two or more days of muscle strengthening activities that work all major muscle groups (legs, hips back, abdomen, chest, shoulders, and arms) could be a modified plank or a push up. Greater levels of activity will provide greater health benefits, but it is important to start to do some form of exercise and build up to the standards. If thirty minutes is too long of a walk, an alternative is to do three ten-minute walks per day. It is important to move more and sit less. Start with small activities and build up to more strenuous ones. All movement, whether aerobic or muscle strengthening, is beneficial. Please consult a doctor before beginning a new exercise regime.

Sleep, sweet sleep.

I have a confession. For most of my life, I have been a person who stayed up late and did not get proper rest. I remember missing sleep as a teenager by talking on the phone late and then doing my homework even later in the night. The next morning, I had difficulty getting out of bed. My mom yelled for me to get up because I had slept too late, and I had to rush to get ready for school. This bad habit continued in college and throughout my life until a few years ago.

Having the ability to stay up longer than the average person has come in handy, especially during my educational career when I had to study for exams and write papers. While working on my doctorate, and writing, at times, I stayed awake all night and then went to work. To be honest, I thought people who had to get their beauty sleep were wimps, but I was wrong. Sleep is important and vital to your health. According to the National, Heart, Lung, and Blood Institute at NIH, adults need 7-8 hours of sleep per night.[4] During sleep, your nervous, circulatory, endocrine, and muscular systems are restored and rejuvenated. Healthy immune functions also occur as a result of adequate sleep. I was not aware of how I was a danger to my mind and body and the people around me by not getting enough sleep.

Sleep deficiency affects healthy brain function, physical health (including weight), and daytime performance and safety. Sleep deprivation effects memory and moods. Your brain restores itself after a good night's sleep, and you can have better memory and positive moods. Lack of sleep over time has been shown to increase the risk of obesity and chronic diseases such as high blood pressure, diabetes, and stroke. Studies show that obesity, diabetes, and high cholesterol are more prevalent among sleepers who have irregular sleep or sleep patterns and hours that greatly vary.[5] Additionally, hormones that trigger whether you feel hungry or full (leptin and ghrelin), do not function properly when you are sleep deprived, and you feel hungrier when you are not well-rested. Getting a good night's sleep will aid in maintaining or losing weight. Functioning well throughout the day may be affected if you do not get proper sleep. Driving while sleep deprived has been compared to driving drunk and puts everyone on the road at risk.

There is a myth that you can *catch up on sleep*. Once the sleep window has passed, it is gone. The sleep deficiency, called *sleep debt* is additive over time. For example, if you lose three hours of sleep over five days, you have a fifteen-hour sleep debt. Taking naps and sleeping more on weekends or other days do not make up for the sleep or replace the benefits you lost. However, a nap can make you feel better.

Sleep is important not only for the reasons mentioned above but also from a spiritual viewpoint. Some people are dreamers. Deep sleep or rapid eye movement (REM) sleep occurs ninety minutes after falling asleep. We dream during this state of sleep. In Job 33:15-16 it clearly states, *"In a dream, in a vision of the night, when deep sleep falleth upon men, in slumberings upon the bed; Then he openeth the ears of men, and sealeth their instruction."* God may give you strategies in your dreams as well as warnings and instructions. If you are not getting adequate sleep, you may be missing out on the physical, mental, and spiritual benefits of sleep.

Summary

Romans 12:1 says," *I beseech you therefore brethren, by the mercies of God that ye present your bodies a living sacrifice, holy, acceptable unto God, which is your reasonable service.* "It is important you worship God with your bodies since you only have one body. Along with eating healthy, exercising and getting proper rest are keys to worshipping God with your bodies. The lack of exercise and sleep increases your risk for chronic diseases such as heart disease and type 2 diabetes. Exercise can improve your health by helping you to lose weight and lower your risk of obesity and disease. As you age, it is important to make sure that you are not sedentary. Walking for thirty minutes five days a week, even if it is in ten-minute increments helps to boost your immune function and ward off diseases.

Sleep is God's way of letting your bodies rest. It helps your organs to recharge, reduce stress, and increase memory and performance during the day. Sleep deprivation can have consequences that affect your physical, emotional, and mental health, and quality of life. When I began to go to bed at a reasonable time and got proper rest, I began to feel more relaxed, dreamed, and I even lost weight.

Exercise and Sleep

Questions for reflection

Exercise

1. Is exercise important for maintaining health? Why?

2. Do you exercise consistently? If yes, how much per week? If no, what prevents you from exercising?

3. What is stopping you from exercising at least ten minutes three times per day (thirty minutes a day)? Five times per week for a total of 150 minutes is ideal.

4. What will help you to exercise regularly?

Tips for Exercise

1. Schedule exercise as you would any other appointment.
2. Take short walks throughout the day.
3. Park further away from your car in the parking lot.
4. Take the stairs instead of the elevator.
5. Join a walking club.
6. Start a walking club.
7. Exercise in your home.

Questions for reflection

Sleep

1. Is sleep important for maintaining health? Why?
2. Can you catch up on my lost sleep?
3. Do you have problems sleeping? Yes or No?
4. Why do you have problems sleeping? If so, what?
5. Do you need to see a health professional to help with your sleep issues?

Tips for sleep

1. Turn off all electronics (TV, phone, computer) one hour before you prepare for bed.
2. Turn off all lights before going to bed.
3. Exercise during the day.
4. Pray and read scripture (not on your phone) before you go to bed.

5. Do not eat three to four hours before you go to bed.

6. Stay away from caffeine five to six hours before bed.

7. Try to go to bed at the same time and wake up at the same time each day.

8. Use a diary or mobile app to track your sleep patterns.

9. If you have sleep issues, go see a sleep doctor.

9

Chief Cook and Bottle Washer

Why You Need a Health Coach

Two are better than one; because they have a good reward for their labour. For if they fall, the one will lift up his fellow: but woe to him that is alone when he falleth; for he hath not another to help him up. Again, if two lie together, then they have heat: but how can one be warm alone? And if one prevail against him, two shall withstand him; and a threefold cord is not quickly broken.

—Ecclesiastes 4:9-12

Growing up in a smaller Southern city, most people knew each other and were friendly. There were no strangers. When we drove around town, everyone waved from their porches. At local grocery stores, folks stopped and talked to one another. We had dinner after church on Sunday then played around the churchyard while our parents talked about their lives. These conversations helped to foster long-term relationships among families. As a child, I felt a sense of accountability to and support from our close-knit Southern community.

Being accountable to someone else is important for achieving goals because it means being responsible for your actions but allowing ourselves to be vulnerable to solicit help. Many of you are the chief cooks and head bottle washers as this chapter is entitled, which means you are responsible for many things on your jobs and in your families. Even with many titles, sometimes you need to be accountable to someone else regarding your health.

Accountability may mean stepping back from some duties to achieve your goals. For example, our family sets goals at the beginning of the year. We hold each other accountable for reaching our goals by checking in at six months to see how we are progressing. If we are having trouble achieving our goals, we discuss and give each other suggestions on how to achieve them. We work together. Having a person to check in with is something we all need to help us accomplish our goals.

We have each other to help achieve our goals. Support is necessary, especially in stressful times. Loneliness and isolation may lead to depression. In the scriptures, the importance of having support is evident.

Two are better than one; because they have a good reward for their labour. For if they fall, the one will lift up his fellow: but woe to him that is alone when he falleth; for he hath not another to help him up. Again, if two lie together, then they have heat: but how can one be warm alone? And if one prevail against him, two shall withstand him; and a threefold cord is not quickly broken. Ecclesiastes 4:9-12

Verse nine describes how two are better than one. Accomplishments occur through partnerships. Verses ten through twelve give more examples of the benefit of support. It says if you fall (literally or figuratively), you will have a partner to lift you up. Verse eleven describes two people who are warm together but cannot be warm when alone. In verse twelve, fighting an enemy (seen or unseen) is more effective with two individuals. A health coach will support and hold you accountable and fight for you to achieve your health goals. Here's how I can help you as a health coach.

What is a health coach?

Health coaching has been proven to modify risk factors for disease in healthy and individuals with common chronic diseases.[1] A health coach wants you to achieve your health goals. Just like a sports coach, a health coach identifies barriers to success and tailors plans for the individual to improve. Health coaches teach and encourage lifestyle changes without judgment or guilt. Health coaches do not promote any specific diet plan or way of eating. They meet the client where they are and help them to make changes that will improve their health. Health coaches are non-physician health professionals who use evidence-based lifestyle management interventions to help the client go from where they are currently in their health goals to where they want to be. A health coach not only supports you but also keeps you accountable.

Why do I need a health coach?

The American Journal of Medicine conducted a survey that found that only 31% of cardiologists and 21% of fellows in-training received no education on nutrition during medical school.[2] This means that some doctors whose specialty is the heart and its functions believe the scientific research that heart disease can be prevented by diet and exercise, but over 60% of them cannot give you advice on what to eat and why you need to eat it. They may give you a pamphlet, but as you can see in this book, a lot more information is necessary to make better food choices. This is where a health coach comes in. They teach and hold their client accountable. Health coaches also have more time than the few minutes a physician allows at an appointment.

The health coach approach is effective because accountability increases your chances of doing what you say because you must report back. Also, social support has been shown to ensure behavioral changes. With diabetes, heart disease, and high blood pressure increasing in America, health coaches may work along with physicians to help the client meet their wellness goals. HBP and type 2 diabetes are largely preventable by losing weight, changing your diet, and exercising.

How do I choose a health coach?

Although health coaches have a variety of academic backgrounds, be sure to look for a health coach that is certified, has been trained in nutrition, and is transparent on how to help achieve health goals. It is okay to ask for proof of certification if there is a lack of confidence with the coach. My practice focuses on making healthy food choices and nutrition, because if you first develop the discipline to eat healthy, this discipline is usually applied to other wellness goals. Health coaches also help the client to reduce stress, get good quality sleep, and develop and maintain an exercise routine.

What services does a health coach provide?

Health coaches help you achieve your health goals by taking an assessment of your health habits and provide an individualized plan. Health coaches provide a variety of services such as individual coaching, pantry makeovers, conduct seminars, workshops, grocery store tours, and online coaching. Some health coaches are personal fitness trainers or gym owners, while others are medical providers. My health coaching practice focuses on making healthy food choices combined with faith to help my clients achieve their goals.

Soon after I received my health coaching credential, I used my new skills on my husband. My husband was a steak and rice man who loved heavily seasoned foods, and he liked sweets. Our health journey began when our family participated in a twenty-one-day Daniel Fast in January two years ago, a temporary eating plan I recommend. The diet is based on how Daniel ate in the Old Testament in the Bible. In this fast, we did not eat meats, sweets, processed foods, or drinks. By not eating these foods, we avoided unhealthy fats and sugars, artificial sweeteners, flavorings, colors, food dyes, added sugars, and we ate limitless fruits and vegetables. The fast also increased our spiritual discipline and faith by focusing on God and seeking His guidance. We studied specific Bible passages for twenty-one days which was the spiritual purpose for the fast. This fast was not a weight loss plan, but we did shed a few pounds. We participated in the Daniel Fast with a local church, so that helped keep our family accountable. The modern-day Daniel Fast has been studied by scientists and was found to reduce blood pressure, significantly reduce LDL cholesterol, and reduce insulin for men and women.[3] Before participating in any fast, please consult with a physician.

Before the Daniel Fast, we followed the Southern eating pattern, regularly ate cookies, snacks, soda, juice, and most types of meat. During the fast, my husband complained about bland food. He thought I was *insulting* him with the healthy and "tasteless" food choices. After the twenty-one day fast ended, we added back a few items in our diet but continued to eat healthier than we did before the fast. After two years, we still ate healthier, and my husband lost fifty-three pounds with the food changes only. It was through modifying the Daniel Fast that I came up with the five steps in this book. When my husband went for a routine doctor's visit, his doctor did not recognize him. He had some health issues like gout that flared up based on what he ate. But he no longer had any major gout attacks for several years, and if he had a mild one, it resolved faster. When my husband decided to take his food choices to another level by not eating chicken (including fried chicken) and beef, I did not know whether to cry or laugh. I had not given up those meats, and I had no idea what I would cook for our meals.

As our family changed our eating patterns, I coached my cousin who lived in another state to change her eating habits. She was a busy mother with five children. We managed to text and talk by phone at least once a week and even while she shopped for groceries. By changing her diet and moderate exercise, she lost twenty-five pounds. Her success was acquiring the knowledge of what to eat and having someone to keep her accountable.

My weight fluctuated for many years (mostly increasing), but using the five steps included in this book, I lost fifteen pounds and kept it off for three years. I will use my coaching knowledge and the five steps to help you achieve your health goals. As a certified health coach, my goal is to provide simple, doable solutions to help you obtain your optimal health and wellness.

Summary

Being raised in a small Southern community, I learned how to depend on but also how to support others. I learned to listen and how to ask the right questions. I use the same style as a health coach in helping you reach your health goals. A health coach is a non-judgmental support and accountability partner who meets you where you are. My practice focuses on making healthy food choices combined with faith. I will provide resources, encouragement, and help to develop healthy habits for life. If you are feeling overwhelmed or lost and would like to change your life, I welcome the opportunity to be your health coach.

Again I say to you, that if two of you shall agree on earth as touching any thing that they shall ask, it will be done for them of my Father which is in heaven.

—*Matthew 18:19*

10

Don't Let the Door Hit Ya Where the Good Lord Split Ya

The Charge

Beloved I wish above all things that thou mayest prosper and be in health, even as thy soul prospereth.

—3 John 2

I was in the grocery store, and my shopping cart was full of healthy foods—strawberries, spinach, plain Greek yogurt, nuts, and water. The customer in the checkout line in front of me said, "I see you are one of those healthy eating people. Why don't you have any snacks in the cart? Go ahead and eat your spinach salad and strawberries. Yuck." We began to have a conversation about health and how foods affect how we feel and how some diseases can be prevented or reversed through diet and exercise. I stressed the importance of eating a healthy diet to prevent diseases or premature death. Even after my twenty second speech, he said he was a Southerner, and he would rather die happy and full of fried chicken and beer than to eat bland food and suffer.

Your eating habits are learned behavior from childhood. You may have poor eating habits because your families may not have known what foods were healthy, and therefore, you ate what your families ate. Many recipes were passed from generation to generation. The Southern style of preparing collard greens is to season with a fatty meat like ham hocks. But collard greens can be seasoned with a leaner meat like turkey or even no meat by using garlic and onions instead. It is important for you to explore healthier ways to cook traditional food.

There are hundreds of diets—Nordic, Paleo, Keto, Dr. Atkins, flexitarian, MIND diet, cabbage and soup, low carb, high carb, high fat, cayenne and lemon juice—do you get the picture? There is no shortage of diets, and a new one is released yearly. There is no one perfect diet. Nowadays, you may be considered part of a clique if you say you are a pescatarian, vegan, vegetarian, flexitarian, or ovo-lactarian. You must choose the best eating plan for your health. I am not a proponent of many diets or eating plans, but if I had to recommend three of them, it would be the traditional African diet, the Mediterranean eating plan, and the DASH diet. The traditional African diet focuses on foods from countries from the continent of Africa such as, colorful fruits and vegetables, fish, poultry, yams, beans, nuts, and whole grain foods and limiting sweets. The Mediterranean eating plan is the way that people eat in Italy, Spain, Greece, and other countries in that region. This diet plan is similar to the traditional African diet because it reduces the risk of heart disease.[1] The diet has also been found to reduce the incidence of Parkinson's and Alzheimer's diseases. The diet focuses on eating fruits and vegetables, fish, and whole grains while limiting red meat. The third diet is the DASH diet mentioned in Chapter 4. This diet was created for people who have high blood pressure. It limits foods that are high in saturated fat, such as fatty meats, full-fat dairy products, and tropical oils such as coconut, palm kernel, and palm oils. More information about the history of DASH diet plan can be found in a book by Thomas Moore, *The DASH Diet for Hypertension: Dietary Approach to Stop Hypertension.*

My testimony with my new family doctor

The medical assistant took my blood pressure, and it was in a normal range. I was little shocked since my blood pressure tends to run high. After all my vitals had been taken, everything was normal. Then the family history questions began.

- Do you have a history of cancer in your family? Yes.
- What types? I explained the types of cancer my parents died of.
- History of strokes? Yes.
- Heart disease? Yes.
- High blood pressure? Yes
- Diabetes? Yes.

I answered yes to almost all the medical history questions. My new primary care physician entered the room.

She asked what brought me in that day. I answered I was there for my annual physical.

She asked if there were any issues I wanted to discuss. When I said no, she proceeded with the exam.

She thanked me, and I replied, "You are welcome."

About thirty seconds went by without discussion, then my doctor asked if I took a multivitamin. When I said no, she suggested I take a multivitamin each day. I asked what brand or type because of all the choices, and my doctor said any over the counter multivitamin would be okay.

That was the experience of my annual physical for the last three years—quick and quiet. However, as a health coach, while I know each person's health status and health journey is different, I want others to prosper and be in good health.

Conclusion

Whether therefore ye eat, or drink, or whatsoever ye do,
do all to the glory of God.

—1 Corinthians 10:31

Growing up my Mama always cooked the holiday ham for our family in a pan that was almost too small for it. I saw my mom forcing the ham in a small pan to cook it. I asked my Mama why she cooked the ham in such a small pan if there were larger pans in the kitchen. My Mama replied, "This is the way my mama used to cook the ham, and it always turns out delicious." I called my grandmama and asked why she cooked the ham in such a small pan, and my grandmama replied, "Sweet grandbaby, I used the small pan because that was the only pan I had." We must examine our Southern food traditions to make sure they are the best foods for us, or are we eating the same foods just like my mother who cooked the ham each year in a pan that was too small?

I know you are wondering, *Where do I start?* Congratulations, you have already started by beginning to examine your Southern food traditions and eating patterns (or any food patterns) by reading this book. You have mastered the three sections of the book—awareness, making healthier choices, and accountability. Growing up as a Southerner was filled with many social events that centered around the church, community, and food. We had a great sense of community and love at these events that I cherish, and it made me who I am today. Unfortunately, some of the food traditions were not good for my health, like frying foods instead of baking or broiling them, adding animal fat to season vegetables, and eating large food portions. Other traditions like eating numerous fresh fruits and vegetables are healthy and should be continued. Hopefully, this book has opened an awareness about the Southern eating pattern and food traditions.

Southerners diagnosed with chronic diseases such as heart disease, diabetes, and hypertension at earlier ages are contributed to a Southern eating plan. As you age, it is important to break bad lifestyle habits, or you will suffer the consequences. 10,000 Americans will turn sixty-five each day from now until the end of 2029, and the overall number of people with multiple chronic diseases will increase greatly. You need to change the statistics and leave a health legacy for your children and grandchildren by giving them the tools to make healthy choices about food.

After I became a certified health coach, several people asked me to write a simple book for Southerners that contained tips anyone could implement to jumpstart their health journey. One friend requested I write the book so her seventy-three-year-old mother would read, and easily understand. Because my weight had gone up and down (mostly up) over the last ten years, I needed simple steps to help maintain my weight so I would not have three sizes of clothes in my closet. I wanted to eat healthy and not be hungry or be in the gym for three hours a day. I wanted to prevent the diseases for which I was at risk and common in my family. I took some time to sort through contradictory health studies to develop simple and doable steps to healthy eating. The five simple steps are:

1) Read your labels.
2) Reduce your sodium.
3) Reduce your sugar.
4) Reduce your portions.
5) Eat more fruits and vegetables.

I suggest before beginning the steps, you should ask God if there are root issues (other than being Southern) that may be causing your unhealthy eating habits. There may be traumatic experiences from childhood which caused unforgiveness, anger, rage, self-rejection, and self-doubt. All these things may spiritually influence your eating habits and patterns and whether you are overweight or have obesity. After you discover your negative emotions, God can set you free. Galatians 5:1 states, "*Stand fast therefore in the liberty wherewith Christ hath made us free and be not entangled again with the yoke of bondage.*"

Next, you can ask God to help you use this book as a guide to change your habits. In Matthew 7:7 it tells you, "*Ask, and it shall be given you; seek and ye shall find; knock and it shall be opened unto you.*" Nothing happens overnight. Your eating habits did not develop overnight. For any change to occur, you must start somewhere. After you examine your eating habits, you can proceed with the five steps.

Another component to maintaining your changes is accountability. Your doctor may tell you that you need to lose weight, and losing 10% of your body weight may make a difference in your health. Unfortunately, many physicians have not been trained to tell you *how* we need to lose weight in terms of your eating patterns. So, after reading this book and implementing the steps, accountability is necessary. Accountability may be getting a health coach or joining a health coaching group.

I want to encourage you to understand if you are breathing, then there is room for improvement and change. Your lifestyle habits may prevent or reverse a disease, which may free you from having to take medication. We are in this together. I, too, have risk factors for disease.

It takes self-discipline to change any habits, including eating habits. Self-discipline is the ability to control one's feelings and overcome one's weaknesses. We need self-discipline to regularly read the word of God, pray, to attend church services, and to worship and praise God. You need the same self-discipline to change your food habits. If you get off track one day or week, you cannot beat yourself up. Instead, you need to get back up and start again the next day. This is like our daily walk with Christ. In the Lord's prayer, Matthew 6:11, it says *"Give us this day our daily bread,"* so each day you have grace and mercy to make it. Take one day at a time to change eating patterns and habits. Let's put your faith in your diet and health. Come take this health journey with me and Him. As we read in 1 Peter 5:7, *"Cast your cares on Him because he careth for you."* I pray this book has been a blessing to you because your health is a matter of life and death.

Appendix A

U.S. Department of Agriculture Pesticide Data Program Report Environmental working group deems the dirtiest produce in 2019. The dirtiest means that the foods that contained the highest level of pesticides after being tested. Each year this report is compiled by the USDA and the Environmental Protection Agency.

Dirty dozen list means the most likely foods to contain a pesticide residue.

1. Strawberries

2. Spinach

3. Kale

4. Nectarines

5. Apples

6. Grapes

7. Peaches

8. Cherries

9. Pears

10. Tomatoes

11. Celery

12. Potatoes

Appendix B

Clean 15 (2019) are the least likely fruits and vegetables to contain a pesticide residue.

1. Avocados

2. Sweet Corn

3. Pineapples

4. Frozen sweet peas

5. Onions

6. Papayas

7. Eggplants

8. Asparagus

9. Kiwis

10. Cabbages

11. Cauliflower

12. Cantaloupes

13. Broccoli

14. Mushrooms

15. Honeydews

Appendix C

Tips on whether a fruit or vegetable is organic.

- On loose fruits and vegetables, read the Price Look Up (PLU) code. If the PLU code has only four numbers, this means that the produce was grown conventionally or traditionally (non-organic) with the use of pesticides. The four numbers are the type of fruit or vegetable we are about to purchase.

- If there are five numbers in the PLU code, and the number starts with "8," this tells us that the item is genetically modified.

- If there are five numbers in the PLU code, and it starts with a "9," the produce is organic.

Endnotes

Introduction

1. Vaccarino, Franco, Gerritsen, T. "Exploring Clergy Self-Care: A New Zealand Study." *The International Journal of Religion and Spirituality in Society*. 3 no.2 (2013) DOI: 10.18848/2154-8633/CGP/v03i02/59264

2. Shikany, James M. Monika M. Safford, P.K. Newby, Ragan W. Durant, Todd M. Brown, Suzanne E. Judd. "Southern Dietary Pattern is Associated with Hazard of Acute Coronary Heart Disease in the Reasons for Geographic and Racial Differences in Stroke (REGARDS) Study." *Circulation 132*, no. 9 (2015):804-14. doi:10.1161/CIRCULATIONAHA.114.014421

3. Baqiyyah N. Conway, Xijing Han, Heather M. Munro, Amy L. Gross, Xiao-Ou Shu, Margaret K. Hargreaves,

Wei Zheng, Alvin C. Powers, William J. Blot. "The obesity epidemic and rising diabetes incidence in a low-income racially diverse southern US cohort." *PLOS ONE*, 2018; 13 (1): e0190993 DOI: 10.1371/journal. pone.0190993

4.   Myers, Candice A. Tim Slack, Stephanie T. Broyles, Steven B. Heymsfield, Timothy S. Church, Corby K. Martin. "Diabetes Prevalence is Associated with Different Community Factors in the Diabetes Belt Versus the Rest of the United States." *Obesity (Silver Spring, Md.) 25* no. 2 (2017): 452-459. doi:10.1002/ oby.21725

Chapter 1

1.   CDC, National Center for Chronic Disease Prevention and Health Promotion. "Chronic Diseases in America." Last reviewed October 23, 2019. https://www.cdc.gov/ chronicdisease/resources/infographic/chronic-diseases. htm

2.   Guiding principles for the care of older adults with multimorbidity: an approach for clinicians. American Geriatrics Society Expert Panel on the Care of Older Adults with Multimorbidity. *Journal of the American Geriatric Society* 60 no.10 E1-E25. (2012): doi: 10.1111/j.1532-5415.2012.04188.

3.   Raghupath, Wullianallur and Viju Raghupathi. "An Empirical Study of Chronic Diseases in the United States: A Visual Analytics Approach to Public Health." *International Journal Environmental Research and Public Health 15* no. 3 (2018): 431. doi: 10.3390/ ijerph15030431

4.   American Association of Retired Persons Chronic Conditions among Older Americans. "Chronic Conditions Among Older Americans." (accessed on 1 January 2020) https://assets.aarp.org/rgcenter/health/beyond_50_hcr_conditions.pdf

5.   Tinker Ann. "How to Improve Patient Outcomes for Chronic Diseases and Comorbidities." (accessed on 30 December 2017) http://www.healthcatalyst.com/wp-content/uploads/2014/04/How-to-Improve-Patient-Outcomes.pdf.

6.   Cunningham, Timothy J., Jane B. Croft, Yong Liu, Hua Lu, Paul I. Eke and Wayne H. Giles, "Vital Signs: Racial Disparities in Age-Specific Mortality Among Blacks or African Americans — United States, 1999–2015." *MMWR Morbidity Mortality Weekly Report* 66 (2017): 444–456. DOI: http://dx.doi.org/10.15585/mmwr.mm6617e1External.

7.   National Institutes of Health, National Institute of Diabetes and Digestive and Kidney Diseases (NIDDK). "Overweight and Obesity Statistics." Last modified August 2017. https://www.niddk.nih.gov/health-information/health-statistics/overweight-obesity

8.   *QuickStats*: Number of Youths Aged 2–19 Years and Adults Aged ≥20 Years with Obesity or Severe Obesity — National Health and Nutrition Examination Survey, 2015–2016. MMWR Morbidity and Mortality Weekly Report (2018);67:966. DOI: http://dx.doi.org/10.15585/mmwr.mm6734a7external icon.

9. Truth for America's Health." The State of Obesity: Better Policies for a Healthier America." (September, 2019). https://www.tfah.org/wp-content/uploads/2019/09/2019ObesityReportFINAL-1.pdf

10. Heron, Melanie. "Deaths: Leading Causes for 2017" *National Vital Statistics Reports 68* no. 6 (2019): https://www.cdc.gov/nchs/data/nvsr/nvsr68/nvsr68_06-508.pdf

11. American Heart Association News. "Heart disease Kills More Southerners than any Other Disease." (2016, November 8) https://newsarchive.heart.org/heart-disease-kills-more-southerners-than-any-other-disease/

12. American Heart Association News." More than 100 million Americans have High Blood Pressure, AHA says. (2018, January 31). https://www.heart.org/en/news/2018/05/01/more-than-100-million-americans-have-high-blood-pressure-aha-says

13. Benjamin, Emelia J., Salim S. Virani, Clifton W. Callaway, Alanna M. Chamberlain, Alexander R. Chang, Susan Cheng, Stephanie E. Chiuve, Mary Cushman, Francesca N. Delling, Rajat Deo et al. "AHA Statistical Report Heart Disease and Stroke Statistics-2018 Update: A Report from the American Heart Association." *Circulation 137* no. e67-e492. (2018): DOI: 10.1161/CIR.0000000000000558

14. Whelton, Paul K., Robert M. Carey, Wilbert S. Aronow, Donald E. Casey Jr., Karen J. Collins, Cheryl Dennison Himmelfarb, Sondra M. DePalma, Samuel Gidding, Kenneth A. Jamerson, Daniel W. Jones et al,. "2017

ACC/AHA/AAPA/ABC/ACPM/AGS/APhA/ASH/ ASPC/NMA/PCNA Guideline for the Prevention, Detection, Evaluation, and Management of High Blood Pressure in Adults: A Report of the American College of Cardiology/American Heart Association Task Force on Clinical Practice Guidelines. "Journal *of the American College of Cardiology 71*, no.19 (2018): DOI: 10.1016/j.jacc.2017.11.006

15. ACC News Story. American College of Cardiology. "New ACC/AHA High Blood Pressure Guidelines Lower Definition of Hypertension." (November 13, 2017)

    https://www.acc.org/latest-in-cardiology/articles /2017/11/08/11/47/mon-5pm-bp-guideline-aha-2017

16. Howard, George, Mary Cushman, Claudia S. Moy, Suzanne Oparil, Paul Muntner, Daniel T. Lackland, Jennifer Manly, Matthew Flaherty, Suzanne E. Judd, Virginia G. Wadley et al. "Association of Clinical and Social with Excess Hypertension Risk in Black Compared with White US Adults." *Journal of the American Medical Association 320* no. 12 (2018): 1338-1348. doi:10.1001/jama.2018.13467

17. Centers for Disease Control and Prevention. *National Diabetes Statistics Report, 2017.* Atlanta, GA: Centers for Disease Control and Prevention, US Department of Health and Human Services; 2017. https://www. cdc.gov/diabetes/data/statistics/statistics-report.html

18. Conway, Baqiyyah N., Xijing Han, Heather M. Munro, Amy L. Gross, Xiao-Ou Shu, Margaret K. Hargreaves, Wei Zheng, Alvin C. Powers, and William J. Blot.

"The obesity epidemic and rising diabetes incidence in a low-income racially diverse southern US cohort." *PLOS ONE* January 11, 2018 doi.org/10.1371/journal. pone.0190993

19. Centers for Disease Control and Prevention. National Diabetes Prevention Program. Last reviewed August 10, 2019 https://www.cdc.gov/diabetes/prevention/index.html

Chapter 2

1. Wiss, David, Nicole Avena & Pedro Rada. "Sugar Addiction: From Evolution to Revolution." *Frontiers in Psychiatry*, 07 November 2018. doi.org/10.3389/fpsyt.2018.00545

2. Merrick, Melissa T, Derek C. Ford, Katie A. Ports, Angie S. Guinn, Jieru Chen, Joanne Klevens, Marilyn Metzler, Christopher M. Jones, Thomas R. Simon, Valerie M. Daniel, Phyllis Ottley, and James A. Mercy, "*Vital Signs:* Estimated Proportion of Adult Health Problems Attributable to Adverse Childhood Experiences and Implications for Prevention — 25 States, 2015–2017. "*Morbidity and Mortality Weekly Report.* 68 no.44 (2019): 999-1005 DOI: http://dx.doi.org/10.15585/mmwr.mm6844e1

3. Stevens, Jane Ellen. Toxic stress from childhood trauma causes obesity, too. ACES too High News. (2012, May 23). https://acestoohigh.com/2012/05/23/toxic-stress-from-childhood-trauma-causes-obesity-too/

4.   Wright, Henry W. A More Excellent Way: Be in Health: Pathways of Wholeness, Spiritual Roots of Disease. Whitaker House, New Kensington, PA 2009

5.   Wade, Terrance J, Deborah D. O'Leary, Kylie S. Dempster, Adam J. MacNeil, Danielle S. Molnar, Jennifer McGrath, and John Cairney. "Adverse childhood experiences (ACEs) and cardiovascular development from childhood to early adulthood: study protocol of the Niagara Longitudinal Heart Study." *BMJ Open* 9 no. 7 (2019): e030339. doi: 10.1136/bmjopen-2019-030339

Chapter 3

1.   Calvo, Trisha. "Key Changes on the New Nutrition Labels" *Consumer Reports*. December 28, 2019. https://www.consumerreports.org/food-labels/key-changes-on-new-nutrition-labels/

2.   FDA. "Nutrition Education Resources & Materials. New and Improved Nutrition Facts Label." https://www.fda.gov/food/food-labeling-nutrition/nutrition-education-resources-materials

3.   U.S. Department of Health and Human Services and U.S. Department of Agriculture. *2015 – 2020 Dietary Guidelines for Americans*. 8th Edition. December 2015. Available at https://health.gov/dietaryguidelines/2015/guidelines/

4.   McManus, Katherine D. "Should I be eating more fiber?" *Harvard Health Blog* (blog). (February 27, 2019). https://www.health.harvard.edu/blog/should-i-be-eating-more-fiber-2019022115927

5. The American Heart Association. "Sugar 101" (July 27, 2018). https://www.heart.org/HEARTORG/ HealthyLiving/HealthyEating/%20HealthyEating/ Sugar-101_UCM_306024_Article.jsp

6. Rippe, James M., and Theodore J. Angelopoulos. "Relationship between Added Sugars Consumption and Chronic Disease Risk factors: Current Understanding." *Nutrients* 8 no. 11 (2016): 697 doi: 10.3390/nu8110697

7. Calvo, Trisha. "Key Changes on the New Nutrition Labels" *Consumer Reports*. December 28, 2019. https://www.consumerreports.org/food-labels/ key-changes-on-new-nutrition-labels/

8. Cozma, Adrian I., John L. Sievenpiper. "The Role of Fructose, Sucrose, and Hi-Fructose Corn Syrup and Diabetes." *European Endocrinology* 10 no. 1 (2014): 51-60. doi: 10.17925/EE.2014.10.01.51

9. Wendorf, Marcia. "High Fructose Corn Syrup and the Obesity Epidemic." March 29, 2019. https:// interestingengineering.com/high-fructose-corn- syrup-and-the-obesity-epidemic

10. Potera, Carol. "Diet and Nutrition: The Artificial Food Dye Blues." *Environmental Health Perspectives* 118 no. 10 (2010): A428 doi: 10.1289/ehp.118-a428

Chapter 4

1. The American Heart Association. "How much sodium should I eat per day?" May 23, 2018. https://www. heart.org/en/healthy-living/healthy-eating/eat-smart/ sodium/how-much-sodium-should-i-eat-per-day

2. Harnack, Lisa J., Mary E. Cogswell, James M. Shikany, Christopher D. Gardner, Cathleen Gillespie, Catherine M. Loria, Xia Zhou, Kemin Yuan and Lyn M. Steffen." Sources of sodium in the U.S. adults from three geographic regions." Circulation (2017): 135: 1775-1783. doi.org/10.1161/CIRCULATIONAHA.116.024446

3. Conis, Elena. "Beware of the hidden salt in chicken." Chicago Tribune (2009, August 11). Accessed on 12 27 2019. http://www.chicagotribune.com/lifestyles/health/chi-tc-health-chicken-donejul06-story.html

4. National Heart, Lung, and Blood Institute; National Institutes of Health; U.S. Department of Health and Human Services. "DASH Eating Plan." Accessed on 12 31 2019 https://www.nhlbi.nih.gov/health-topics/dash-eating-plan

Chapter 5

1. Yang, Quanhe, Zefeng Zhang, Edward W. Gregg, Dana Flanders, Robert Merritt and Frank B. Hu. "Added Sugar Intake and Cardiovascular Diseases Mortality Among US Adults." *JAMA Internal Medicine 4* no. 174 (2014): 516-524. doi:10.1001/jamainternmed.2013.13563

2. Knüppel, Anika, Martin J. Shipley, Clare H. Llewellyn, and Eric J. Brunner. Sugar intake from sweet food and beverage, common mental disorder and depression: prospective findings from the Whitehall II study." *Scientific Reports 7* no. 6287 (2017): 1-10. doi:10.1038/s41598-017-05649-7

3. Guo, Xuguang, Yikung Park, Neal D. Freedman, Rashmi Sinha, Albert R. Hollenbeck, Aaron Blair

and Honglei Chen. "Sweetened Beverages, Coffee, and Tea and Depression Risk among Older US Adults." *PLOS ONE, 9* no. 4 (2014): e94715 doi.org/10.1371/journal.pone.0094715

4. Wiss, David, Nicole Avena & Pedro Rada. "Sugar Addiction: From Evolution to Revolution." *Frontiers in Psychiatry,* 07 November 2018. doi.org/10.3389/fpsyt.2018.00545

5. Vasselli, Joseph R., Philip J. Scarpace, Ruth B. S. Harris, and William A. Banks. "Dietary Components in the Development of Leptin Resistance." *Advances in Nutrition,* 4 no. 2 (2013): 164–175. doi.org/10.3945/an.112.0031

6. Aragno, Manuela and Raffaella Mastrocola. "Dietary Sugars and Endogenous Formation of Advanced Glycation Endproducts: Emerging Mechanisms of Disease." *Nutrients, 9* no. 4 (2017): 385. doi.org/10.3390/nu9040385

7. Katta, Rajani and Samir P. Desai. "Diet and Dermatology: The Role of Dietary Intervention in Skin Disease." *The Journal of Clinical and Aesthetic Dermatology* 7 no. 7 (2014): 1-15.

8. Johnson, Rachel K., Lawrence J. Appel, Michael Brands, Barbara V. Howard, Michael Lefevre, Robert H. Lustig, Frank Sacks, Lyn M. Steffen, Judith Wylie-Rosett on behalf of the American Heart Association Nutrition Committee of the Council on Nutrition, Physical Activity, and Metabolism and the Council on Epidemiology and Prevention. "Dietary sugar intake and cardiovascular health a scientific statement from the American

Heart Association." *Circulation, 120* (2009): 1011-1020. DOI: 10.1161/CIRCULATIONAHA.109.192627

9. The American Heart Association. "Sugar 101" (July 27, 2018). https://www.heart.org/HEARTORG/ HealthyLiving/HealthyEating/%20HealthyEating/ Sugar-101_UCM_306024_Article.jsp

10. Mock, Kaitlin, Sundus Lateef, Vagner A. Benedito and Janet C. Tou. High-Fructose Corn Syrup-55 consumption alters hepatic Lipid Metabolism and Promotes Triglyceride Accumulation" The *Journal of Nutritional Biochemistry* 39 (2017): 32-39 doi.org/10.1016/j. jnutbio.2016.09.010

11. Chung, Mei, Jianto Ma, Samantha Berger, Joseph Lau and Alice H. Lichtenstein. "Fructose, high-fructose corn syrup, sucrose, and nonalcoholic fatty liver disease or indexes of liver health: a systematic review and meta-analysis." *The American Journal of Clinical Nutrition* 100 no. 3 (2014): 833-849. doi.org/10.3945/ ajcn.114.086314

12. Gardner, Christopher, Judith Wylie-Rosett, Samuel S. Gidding, Lyn M. Steffen, Rachel K. Johnson, Diane Reader, Alice H. Lichtenstein, and on behalf of the American Heart Association Nutrition Committee of the Council on Nutrition, Physical Activity and Metabolism, Council on Arteriosclerosis, Thrombosis and Vascular Biology, Council on Cardiovascular Disease in the Young, and the American Diabetes Association."Nonnutritive sweeteners: current use and health perspectives: a scientific statement from the American Heart Association and the American

Diabetes Association *Diabetes Care 35* no. 8 (2012): 1798-1808. doi.org/10.2337/dc12-9002

13. Mayo Clinic. "Artificial sweeteners and other sugar substitutes." Accessed December 26, 2019 https://www.mayoclinic.org/healthy-lifestyle/nutrition-and-healthy-eating/in-depth/artificial-sweeteners/art-20046936

Chapter 6

1. American Heart Association. "Heavy Meals May Trigger Heart Attacks." ScienceDaily. www.sciencedaily.com/releases/2000/11/001120072759.htm (accessed February 2, 2020).

2. National Heart, Lung, and Blood Institute; National Institutes of Health; U.S. Department of Health and Human Services. Home Health Information for the Public Educational Campaigns & Programs *We Can!* Eat Right. "Serving Sizes and Portions: Portion Distortions" Last updated September 30, 2013. https://www.nhlbi.nih.gov/health/educational/wecan/eat-right/distortion.htm

3. Bouvard, Véronique, Dana Loomis, Kathryn Z. Guyton, Yann Grosse, Fatiha El Ghissassi, Lamia Benbrahim-Talla, Neela Guha, Heidi Mattock and Kurt Straif on behalf of the International Agency for Research on Cancer Monograph Working Group. "Carcinogenicity of Consumption of Red and Processed Meat." *The Lancet Oncology* 16 no.16 (2015): 1599-1600. doi: 10.1016/S1470-2045(15)00444-1

4.	Campbell, T. Colin, Thomas Campbell II. *The China Study: Startling Implications for Diet, Weight loss and Long Term Health.* Dallas: Benbella, 2006.

5.	Wyness, Laura. "The Role of Red Meat in the Diet: Nutrition and Health Benefits." *Proceedings of the Nutrition Society* 75 no. 3 (2016): 227-232. doi: 10.1017/S0029665115004267

6.	Cross, Amanda J., Leah M. Ferucci, Adam Risch, Barry I. Graubard, Mary H. Ward, Yikyung Park, Albert R. Hollenbeck, Arthur Schatzkin and Rashmi Sinha. "A Large Prospective Study of Meat Consumption and Colorectal Cancer Risk: An Investigation of Potential Mechanism Underlying this Association." *Cancer Research* 70 no. 6 (2010): 2406-2414. DOI: 10.1158/0008-5472.CAN-09-3929

7.	United States Department of Agriculture. "Choose-MyPlate"(n.d.). https://www.choosemyplate.gov/WhatIsMyPlate

Chapter 7

1.	Eman, Alissa and Gordon A. Ferns. "Dietary fruits and vegetables and cardiovascular risk." *Critical Reviews in Food Science and Nutrition.* 57 no. 9 (2017): 1950-1962 DOI:10.1080/10408398.2015.1040487

2.	The American Heart Association. (2019). Fruits and vegetables serving sizes. https://www.heart.org/en/healthy-living/healthy-eating/add-color/fruits-and-vegetables-serving-sizes

3.	McManus, Katherine D., "Should I be eating more fiber?" Harvard Health (blog), February 27, 2019, https://www.

health.harvard.edu/blog/should-i-be-eating-more-fibe
r-2019022115927

4. Reynolds, Andrew, Jim Mann, John Cummings, Nicola
    Winter MDiet, Evelyn Mete MDiet, Lisa Te Morenga.
    "Carbohydrate Quality and Human Health: A Series
    of Systematic Reviews and Meta-Analyses." *The Lancet
    393* no.10170 (2019) :434-445.

    doi.org/10.1016/S0140-6736(18)31809-9

Chapter 8

1. Choi, Karmen. W., Chia-Yen Chen, Murray B. Stein,
    Yann C. Klimentidis, Min-Jun Wang, Karestan C.
    Koenen, Jordan W. Smoller, for the Major Depressive
    Disorder Working Group of the Psychiatric Genomics
    Consortium. "Assessment of bidirectional relationships
    between physical activity and depression among adults:
    A 2-sample mendelian randomization study." *JAMA
    Psychiatry 76*, no.4 (2019): 399-408. doi:10.1001/
    jamapsychiatry.2018.4175

2. Legey, Sandro, Filipe Aquino, Murilo Khede Lamego,
    Flavia Paes, Antonio Egidio Nardi, Geraldo Maran-
    hao Neto, Gioia Mura, Federoca Sancassiani, Nuno
    Rocha, Eric Murillo-Rodriguez and Sergio Mach-
    ado. "Relationship Among Physical Activity Level,
    Mood and Anxiety States and Quality of Life in
    Physical Education Students." *Clinical Practice and
    Epidemiology in Mental Health* 13 (2017): 82-91. DOI:
    10.2174/1745017901713010082

3. U.S. Department of Health and Human Services.
    *Physical Activity Guidelines for Americans, 2nd edi-
    tion.* Washington, DC: U.S. Department of Health

and Human Services; 2018. https://health.gov/paguidelines/second-edition/

4. National Heart, Lung, and Blood Institute; National Institutes of Health; U.S. Department of Health and Human Services. *Sleep Deprivation and Deficiency.* https://www.nhlbi.nih.gov/health-topics/sleep-deprivation-and-deficiency

5. Huang, Tianyi, and Susan Redline. "Cross-sectional and Prospective Associations of Actigraphy-Assessed Sleep Regularity with Metabolic Abnormalities: The Multi-Ethnic Study of Atherosclerosis." *Diabetes Care.* 42 no. 8 (2019): 1422-1429. doi: https:org/10.2337/dc19-0596

Chapter 9

1. Gordon, Neil, Richard D. Salmon, Brenda S. Wright, George C. Faircloth, Kevin S. Reid and Terri L. Gordon. "Clinical Effectiveness of Lifestyle Health Coaching." *American Journal of Lifestyle Medicine.* 11 no. 2 (2017): 153-166.

2. Devries, Stephen, Arthur Agatson, Monica Aggarwal, Karen E. Aspry, Caldwell B. Esselstyn, Penny Kris-Etherton, Michael Miller, James O'Keefe, Emilio Ros, Anne K. Rzeszut, Beth A. White, Kim A. Williams, Andrew Freeman. "A Deficiency of Nutrition Education and Practice in Cardiology." *The American Journal of Medicine.* 130 no. 11 (2017) :1298-1305 doi: 10.1016/j.amjmed.2017.04.043

3. Bloomer, Richard J., Mohammad M. Kabir, Robert E. Canale, John F. Trepanowski, Kate E. Marshall, Tyler M. Farney and Kelley G. Hammond. "Effect of a 21-day

Daniel Fast on Metabolic and Cardiovascular Disease Risk Factors in Men and Women." *Lipids in health and disease* 9 no. 94. (2010). doi:10.1186/1476-511X-9-94.

Chapter 10

1. Widmer, R. Jay A, Andreas Flammer, Lilach O. Lerman and Amir Lerman. "The Mediterranean Diet, its Components, and Cardiovascular Disease." *The American Journal of Medicine* 128 no. 3 (2015): 229-238. doi. org/10.1016/j.amjmed.2014.10.014

About the Author

Dr. Jennifer Whitmon is an author, health coach and speaker who focuses on teaching individuals how to improve health through simple changes. From her humble beginnings in Gadsden, Alabama, Dr. Whitmon has learned the importance of serving others. After moving to Atlanta, Georgia as a young adult, Dr. Whitmon worked in the religious and secular communities in metropolitan Atlanta neighborhoods, teaching students and families in community programs. She has worked successfully with small and large audiences, including non-profits, businesses, schools, colleges, universities, and churches in the Atlanta metropolitan area, and Southeastern United States. For over twenty years, she has inspired and educated individuals to make better choices regarding their health and faith. Dr. Whitmon holds a Bachelor of Science degree in Biology, Master of Arts degree in Science Education and a Doctorate in Health Science with a concentration in global health. She is a veteran, and lives in Georgia with her husband John and daughter.

Connect with Dr. Whitmon at
www.drjenniferwhitmon.com

Put That Fried Chicken Down

Are you a true Southerner?

What are your eating habits?

Why do you eat the way you do?

Take the Free Assessment:
Get Your Score

Experience a Free Thirty-Minute Consultation
Start Changing Your Habits Now

Sign-Up for the Online Course—Put That Fried Chicken Down
Explore More of the Five Simple Steps

Put That Fried Chicken Down: Online Course

Will help you:
- Understand what's in your food and not be fooled by labels and ingredients
- Avoid high sodium and high sugar foods
- Reduce your food portions
- Eat more fruits and vegetables
- Make better food choices at restaurants

What you will learn:
- Detailed label reading information
- Greenwashing of foods
- Healthy foods you want to eat
- Toxic foods to avoid.
- Health benefits of various fruits
- Health benefits of various vegetables

What people are saying:
- "I lost weight and have information for my family."
- "I didn't know eating healthy was so easy."
- "Thanks for simplifying healthy eating."
- "I feel lighter when I follow the five steps."

What to do:
Visit to learn more about the course and to receive your free gifts.
Gift #1: Healthy Food Swaps for Southerners
Gift #2: Southern Food Hacks
Ready to get started? Visit www.drjenniferwhitmon.com today!

Why we know you will love it:
This a cost-effective way to jumpstart the eating plan. The five simple steps will begin a lifestyle of better eating habits.

www.drjenniferwhitmon.com

Made in the USA
Columbia, SC
20 November 2020

24996823R00085